Queen Elizabeth Hospital

D0270770

100 Clinical Cases
and
OSCEs in Surgery

DATE DUE

			PRINTED IN U.S.A.

PRINTED IN U.S.A.

100 Clinical Cases and OSCEs in Surgery

Noel J Aherne
Enda McDermott
Arnold D K Hill

Department of Surgery
St Vincent's University Hospital
Elm Park
Dublin 4

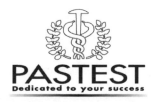

PASTEST
Dedicated to your success

© 2004 PASTEST Ltd
Egerton Court
Parkgate Estate
Knutsford
Cheshire
WA16 8DX

Telephone: 01565 752000

All rights reserved. No part of this publication may be reproduced, stored in a
retrieval system, or transmitted, in any form or by any means, electronic,
mechanical, photocopying, recording or otherwise without the prior permission of the
copyright owner.

First published 2004

ISBN: 1 904627 00 5

A catalogue record for this book is available from the British Library.

The information contained within this book was obtained by the authors from reliable
sources. However, while every effort has been made to ensure its accuracy, no
responsibility for loss, damage or injury occasioned to any person acting or refraining
from action as a result of information contained herein can be accepted by the
publishers or authors.

PasTest Revision Books and Intensive Courses
PasTest has been established in the field of postgraduate medical education since
1972, providing revision books and intensive study courses for doctors preparing for
their professional examinations.

Books and courses are available for the following specialties:
MRCGP, MRCP Parts 1 and 2, MRCPCH Parts 1 and 2, MRCPsych, MRCS, MRCOG Parts
1 and 2, DRCOG, DCH, FRCA, PLAB Parts 1 and 2

For further details contact:
PasTest, Freepost, Knutsford, Cheshire WA16 7BR
Tel: 01565 752000   Fax: 01565 650264
www.pastest.co.uk   enquiries@pastest.co.uk

Text prepared by Carnegie Book Production, Lancaster
Printed and bound by Cromwell Press Ltd, Wiltshire

Contents

Gastrointestinal disorders

Thoracic disorders

General

Urology

Endocrine disorders

Vascular disorders

Musculoskeletal disorders

Hepatobiliary disorders

Introduction

This book addresses the needs of undergraduate medical students who are sitting the OSCE component of their surgical finals. Objectively Structured Clinical Examinations (OSCEs) are becoming more common in undergraduate exams. Their benefit is that they provide objectivity to the assessment of the candidate's ability in a practical environment.

The 100 cases provide a reasonable spectrum of the typical cases seen in final surgery OSCE exams. The book has been divided into the following sections: gastrointestinal, general lumps and skin disorders, urology, endocrine, vascular, musculoskeletal, and hepatobiliary disease. The structure of the book has been written to help the student to identify the core knowledge required in each area, and what points might be had in a discussion with the examiners. It also offers points on advanced issues for ambitious students and those aiming for the MRCS and AFRCSI.

The editors are members of The Department of Surgery at St Vincent's University Hospital. They have a long cumulative history as examiners in University College Dublin. The editors hope that this book you will keep this book and use it often throughout your undergraduate career and beyond. We would like to acknowledge the support of our Head of Department, Professor Niall O'Higgins in writing this book.

Arnold D K Hill, 2004

Abbreviations

AAAs	Abdominal aortic aneurisms
ABI	Ankle-brachial index
ACE	Angiotensin-converting nerve
ADL	Activities of daily living
ALT	Alanine aminotransferase
APC	Adenomatus polyposis coli
APR	Abdomino-perineal resection
AST	Aspartate aminotransferase
ATLS	Advanced trauma life support
BCC	Basal-cell carcinoma
CCA	Common carotid artery
CVA	Cerebrovascular accident
CLO	Campylobacter-like organism
CT	Computed tomography
DVT	Deep vein thrombosis
EMG	Electromyography
ERCP	Endoscopic retrograde
FOB	Faecal occult blood
HLA	Human leukocyte nerve
HPOA	Hypertrophic pulmonary osteoarthropathy
ICA	Internal carotid artery
IPAA	Ileal pouch anal anastomosis
IVC	Inferior vena cava
MNG	Multinodular goitre
MODS	Multiple organ dysfunction syndrome
PICC	Peripherally inserted central catherters
RIND	Reversible carotid artery
RLN	Recurrent laryngeal nerve
RP	Raynaud's phenomenon
SCC	Squamous-cell carcinoma
SCM	Sternocleiodmastoid
SEPS	Subcutaneous endoscopic perforator
TIA	Transient ischaemic attack
TRAM	Transverse rectus abdominus muscle
TSH	Thyroid-stimulating hormone
VWF	Vibration white finger

Gastrointestinal disorders

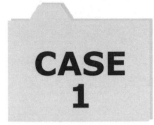

CASE 1

Abdominal examination

Examine this man's abdomen.

🔍 The examination

The examination of the abdomen is common in OSCE exams, as it is a relatively standardised aspect of the clinical examination. Remember the following strategy:

- introduction
- exposure
- position
- inspection/palpation/percussion/auscultation
- extras.

Exposure should be adequate for the examination you wish to perform, and you should be as concerned for the patient's dignity as for your clinical examination. You may begin your examination with the hands, eyes, mouth, neck and trunk, or you may be directed to examine the abdomen specifically.

Wash your hands. Expose the patient to the symphysis pubis, keeping the external genitalia covered. Position the patient as close to the horizontal as they can tolerate, and place a pillow under their head.

Inspect the abdomen from the end of the couch and look for any general abnormalities, such as cachexia, jaundice and pallor. Look for symmetry of the abdomen and its shape. Is it flat, distended or scaphoid? Is the asymmetry global or localised? Look closely for sinuses, scars, fistulae and distended veins. What is the respiratory rate? Confirm this from the right-hand side of the patient, while kneeling.

Ask the patient if they have any pain or discomfort, and palpate from the patient's right side while looking directly at their face. Assess whether there is tenderness, guarding or rebound tenderness present on light palpation. Organomegaly and the presence of masses are best detected by deep palpation.

If you find a mass, apply your basic principles of description:

- site
- size
- shape
- surface
- edge
- consistency
- fluctuation
- fluid thrill
- resonance
- pulsatility.

Now palpate the liver and spleen, and ballot the kidneys as shown in Case 57.

Percussion is probably best reserved for the presence of hepatomegaly, splenomegaly, suspected ascites or intra-abdominal masses. You should be prepared to percuss the organs if requested to do so.

Auscultate for bowel sounds in the left iliac fossa. Auscultate along the course of the aorta, the renal arteries, the iliac arteries and over the liver for bruits.

Complete your examination by feeling the supraclavicular and inguinal regions for lymphadenopathy. Palpate the hernial orifices (external inguinal ring, umbilicus and femoral canal) at rest and while the patient is coughing. Examine the femoral pulses and state that you would like to examine the external genitalia and the urine and perform a digital rectal examination to complete the abdominal examination.

CASE
1

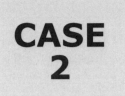

CASE 2

Colostomy

You are shown a patient with a colostomy.

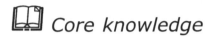 *Core knowledge*

Recognition of a colostomy is based on the following:

- location of stoma in abdominal quadrants, usually left iliac fossa
- if there is only one lumen, it is an end colostomy; if there are two, it is a loop colostomy
- stoma flush with skin
- contents of colostomy bag – more solid than with ileostomy.

Discussion points

Complications of stoma

- Retraction, prolapse, herniation, psychosexual problems (retraction and prolapse are more likely to occur in transverse loop colostomies than in end colostomies or in ileostomies).

Indications for stoma

- Temporary: perforation as in Hartman's procedure (removal of the sigmoid colon due to perforation or obstruction by benign or malignant disease with subsequent exteriorisation of the descending colon and oversewing shut of the rectal stump within the pelvis).
- Permanent: this may occur in abdomino-perineal resection (APR) for ultra-low rectal cancers which are not amenable to colo-anal or colorectal anastomosis.

Gastrointestinal disorders

🎓 *Advanced issues*

- Siting of stoma where it is visible to the patient, away from bony prominences and skin creases. Tell the examiner about involvement of the stomatherapist to aid the patient pre-operatively and also post-operatively (to choose appliances).

- Stoma reversal is desirable in those patients who are fit for re-operation. However, although many patients have a defunctioning colostomy temporarily in the first instance, they may be unfit for restoration of bowel continuity subsequently.

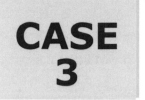

CASE 3

Ileostomy

You are shown a patient with an end ileostomy.

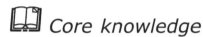

Core knowledge

Recognition of an ileostomy is based on the following:

- location of stoma in abdominal quadrants, usually right iliac fossa
- if there is only one lumen, it is an end ileostomy; if there are two, it is a loop ileostomy
- stoma spouted above skin level
- contents of ileostomy bag – more fluid-like than with colostomy.

Discussion points

- Ileostomy contents are rich in proteolytic and digestive intestinal content, which is potentially harmful to the skin. The ileostomy spout is designed to prevent skin irritation.
- Complications of ileostomies include fluid and electrolyte depletion due to high-volume fluid loss, as well as the complications listed for colostomies.
- Terminal ileal loss may have nutritional implications, such as vitamin B_{12} deficiency or malnutrition due to short bowel syndrome.

Indications for stoma

- Temporary or defunctioning (loop) ileostomy: for example, this may be used after fashioning of an ileo-anal pouch (restorative proctocolectomy) in patients with ulcerative colitis.
- Permanent: following an abdominoperineal resection.

CASE 3

Gastrointestinal disorders

🎓 *Advanced issues*

- Indications for a defunctioning ileostomy in protecting an anastomosis.
- Metabolic derangements with loss of bile salts predisposing to gallstones after ileostomy.

**CASE
3**

CASE 4

Ileal conduit

You are shown a patient with an ileal conduit.

Ileal conduits are the most common form of urinary diversion procedure (urostomy) performed in the UK and Ireland. They are formed by attaching the ureters to one end of an isolated loop of ileum which has been resected. There is no reservoir function, and the result is an incontinent ostomy which fills continuously with urine.

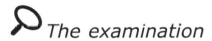

The examination

On inspection, you will see a stoma in the right iliac fossa, commonly with large amounts of clear fluid. There is no spout and the contents are usually clear. The stoma is flush with the skin. There may be associated scars in the lower abdomen from previous bladder surgery or a transverse laparotomy (if the surgery was performed while the patient was a child).

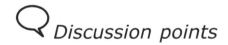

Discussion points

In ileal conduits the urine passes through an ileal segment. Therefore gut bacteria may colonise the ureters, resulting in ascending urinary tract infections and renal infections. Ask the patient about symptoms of urinary tract infections and pyelonephritis.

An alternative to an ileal conduit is a continent urinary ostomy that utilises a valve mechanism which allows the patient either to self-catheterise or to empty the urine manually into a receptacle. One example is a Bendrassik nipple valve.

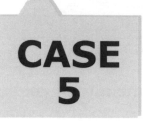

Gastrointestinal disorders

CASE 5

Inguinal hernia

Examine this man's groin for an inguinal hernia.

A hernia is a protrusion of a viscus or part of a viscus through the wall of the space that contains it.

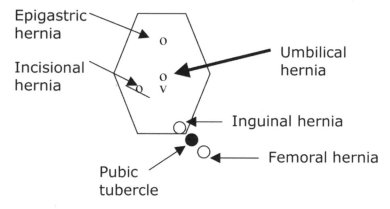

Fig 1 Types of abdominal hernia

The inguinal ligament lies between the anterior superior iliac spine and the pubic tubercle. The pubic tubercle is easy to find if you locate the symphysis pubis and slide your fingers laterally. The inguinal ligament is the lower edge of the aponeurosis of the external oblique muscle. Above this, the fibres of the aponeurosis divide at the pubis to form the external inguinal ring. Below this, the lowermost fibres of the internal oblique muscle rise from the lateral third of the inguinal ligament and arc medially. At the edge of the rectus abdominis, they join with the aponeurosis of the transversus abdominis muscle to form the front of the rectus sheath. Here the common fibres are termed the conjoint tendon.

The space beneath the arc of the internal oblique muscles is not very strong, and is filled with flimsy transversalis fascia. This is the weak spot of the inguinal region, and it is the point where indirect inguinal hernias develop. The inferior epigastric artery runs upward and medially towards the rectus sheath. The internal inguinal ring, where the vas deferens and testicular artery pass through, is lateral to the epigastric artery.

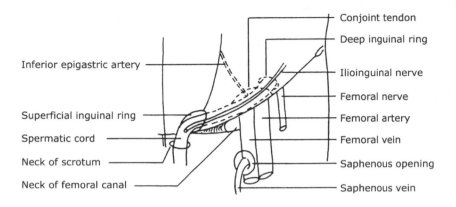

Fig 2 Anatomy of the inguinal canal

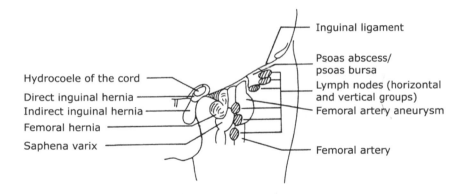

Fig 3 Swellings below the inguinal ligament

Direct inguinal hernias occur on the other side of the inferior epigastric vessels (ie the more medial side) and appear through the back of the posterior wall. As the vas deferens enters the inguinal canal, it first acquires coverings from the transversalis fascia (the internal spermatic fascia), further down it acquires the cremaster muscle and the cremasteric fascia from the internal oblique muscle, and finally it acquires the external spermatic fascia from the external oblique aponeurosis.

As the sac of an indirect inguinal hernia passes down alongside the vas deferens, it lies inside these three coverings and is directed down into the scrotum. In contrast, the direct inguinal hernia begins more medially than this and is separate from the cord structures. Direct inguinal hernias rarely extend into the scrotum.

**CASE
5**

℘ The examination

Direct the patient with regard to exposure and obtain permission to examine him. Expose the patient from the umbilicus to the knees. Any hernia that is visible in the supine position will be more obvious when the patient is standing. However, there is no doubt that the anatomy is easier to define when the patient is lying down, especially if they are obese.

Some of the differential diagnoses in this case include femoral hernias, lymph nodes, femoral aneurysms or saphena varix, and abnormalities of the cord such as hydrocoele and cord lipoma. Therefore it is important that you are certain this lump comes from above the inguinal ligament.

Inspect the patient for scars or an obvious lump. If the hernia is obvious, then palpate it.

If you can demonstrate the origin of the swelling above the inguinal ligament, this is an important finding. Can you get above it? If you can, it is probably a scrotal swelling. Examine the scrotum. Does it have a cough impulse? Is it inguinal or inguinoscrotal? Can it be controlled by taxis at the deep inguinal ring?

With the patient standing, place one hand on the small of his back to support him, and use the other hand to assess the lump under the following headings:

- site
- shape
- size
- tension
- temperature
- tenderness
- contents
- cough impulse
- reducibility.

Complete your examination by auscultating for bowel sounds and examining the other side (around 20% of inguinal hernias are bilateral). Tell the examiner that you would like to ask about predisposing factors such as cough, lifting and altered bowel habit, and to examine the abdomen for any cause of raised intra-abdominal pressure.

CASE 5

$\bigcirc$ *Discussion points*

The differentiation between indirect and direct inguinal hernia does not alter the type of surgical repair, but examiners always ask about this. Indirect inguinal hernias arise in the abdomen and traverse the deep inguinal ring, through the canal, and can be inguinoscrotal. Direct inguinal hernias emerge through a weakness in the posterior wall of the canal and are outside the spermatic cord. They rarely enter the scrotum.

The most common type of hernia repair, namely the Liechtenstein repair, involves placing a polypropylene mesh over the defect and then suturing it in place. This can also be done laparoscopically, using either a transabdominal or a totally extraperitoneal approach.

The contents of the spermatic cord are best remembered in threes:

- the three arteries – the testicular artery, the cremasteric artery and the artery to the vas deferens
- the three nerves – the ilioinguinal nerve, the cremasteric branch of the genitofemoral nerve, and the T10 sympathetic nerve
- the three other structures – the vas, the pampiniform venous plexus and the draining lymph nodes.

The complications of hernia repair are urinary retention, bruising and haematoma formation. These can occur in up to 10% of cases. Pain is usually transient, but up to 5% of patients can experience persistent pain, possibly due to inguinodynia or nerve entrapment. The recurrence rate should be less than 1%.

CASE
5

Gastrointestinal disorders

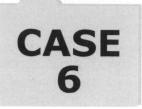

CASE 6

Femoral hernia

Examine this woman's groin for a femoral hernia.

A femoral hernia is a protrusion of extraperitoneal fat, peritoneum and sometimes bowel through the femoral canal. These hernias have a high incidence of strangulation because the borders of the canal are rigid on three sides. Femoral hernias are more common in elderly women, but are not as common as inguinal hernias. They are often bilateral.

๏ The examination

Femoral hernias are repaired as soon as they are diagnosed, so if there is a case on for an examination, it is likely that the patient is symptomatic. Examine the patient while they are lying down, and define the anatomy of the groin, noting the anterior superior iliac spine (ASIS), the pubic tubercle and the groin crease. The hernia usually appears as a visible bulge in the groin crease, but will be below the inguinal ligament, medial to the femoral pulse. Inspect the patient for scars, as the commonest reason for development of a femoral hernia is the repair of an adjacent inguinal hernia.

Assess as you would for any lump, noting the features of a spherical lump with a well-defined edge and smooth consistency. It will not be fluctuant and does not usually have a cough impulse. Femoral hernias are rarely reducible.

Femoral hernias are often bilateral, so examine the other side. The neck of these hernias is below and lateral to the pubic tubercle, in contrast to the inguinal hernia, whose neck is above and medial to the pubic tubercle.

Q Discussion points

Differential diagnosis

- Inguinal hernia
- Lymph nodes
- Saphena varix
- Ectopic testes
- Psoas abscess
- Lipoma.

Inguinal v femoral hernia

Inguinal	Femoral
Above and medial to pubic tubercle	Below and lateral to pubic tubercle
Soft to palpation	Firm to palpation
Resonant to percussion	Dull
May hear bowel sounds	No bowel sounds

With regard to the anatomy of the femoral canal, the femoral nerve lies laterally, with the artery sandwiched between it and the vein, which lies medially. The vein may be compressed if the repair of a hernia is too tight.

Surgery is indicated for all femoral hernias, as the risk of strangulation is high. This can be achieved with a low approach (the commonest type), in which the sac is excised and the canal closed. This is the best approach, but it risks compression of the femoral vein from an overtight repair. Other approaches are a McEvedy repair or a high inguinal repair, which lead to an unacceptably high rate of recurrent inguinal hernias.

CASE 6

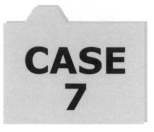

CASE 7

Umbilical hernia

Examine this man's abdomen for an umbilical hernia.

Umbilical hernias are relatively common and are really a collection of hernias. They can be congenital or acquired umbilical, or paraumbilical. The paraumbilical type is most common.

🔍 The examination

Acquired umbilical hernias are uncommon, and you are therefore unlikely to see one in an exam. They appear in the centre of the umbilicus and, importantly, the umbilical skin is attached to them. There will be a defect in the umbilical wall, which will become apparent once the hernia is reduced. They have a cough impulse and many of them contain bowel. They are caused by raised intra-abdominal pressure, so look for a cause after you have defined the hernia. If the neck of the hernia is wide, they are unlikely to strangulate.

Paraumbilical hernias are far more common, and are more likely to be found in an exam. They are more common in obese people, especially women. The defect in the linea alba is adjacent to the umbilicus, the skin is not attached to the sac, and the main prominence of the hernia is to the side of the umbilicus. Most of these patients are obese and complain of pain or a palpable lump. They may give a history of symptoms of intermittent intestinal obstruction.

Palpate the hernial sac. Most contain omentum and will be firm to the touch. If the hernial sac is soft and resonant to percussion, it may contain bowel. Attempt to reduce it. Most will reduce easily, but if it will not reduce then the neck of the sac may be very tight or the contents may be adherent.

Hernias are often multiple, so offer to examine the rest of the abdomen.

Q *Discussion points*

The risk of strangulation in paraumbilical hernias is increased if they contain bowel and if the neck of the sac is narrow. Omentum can also become strangulated, in which case the patient will have severe abdominal pain but no intestinal obstruction.

The repair of umbilical hernias is usually undertaken using a Mayo repair (named after the brothers William and Charles Mayo, founders of the Mayo Clinic). This involves opening and excising the sac, and then suturing the lower edge of the rectus to the upper edge and overlapping the repair.

CASE
7

Gastrointestinal disorders

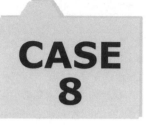

CASE 8   Epigastric hernia

Examine this man's abdomen for an epigastric hernia.

These are small protrusions of extraperitoneal fat that appear in a defect in the linea alba somewhere along a line from the xiphisternum to the umbilicus. The patient usually complains of pain, which may be made worse by eating. These hernias do not usually reduce, and can cause symptoms while they are still very small.

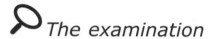

The examination

Direct the patient and obtain adequate exposure as before. The patient will often complain of pain in the epigastric region. Ask them to localize the swelling for you. Raise the intra-abdominal pressure either by placing the chin to the chest (Fothergill's test) or by asking the patient to cough. The swelling may be difficult to find and may require repeated manoeuvres.

On palpation, estimate the size of the hernial defect and assess whether it is reducible or not. Offer to perform a full abdominal examination. Finally, ask about symptoms such as epigastric pain (that is made worse by eating), early satiety or symptoms of reflux.

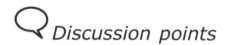

Discussion points

The process of repair is similar to that for umbilical hernias. The sac is excised completely and the linea alba defect is repaired.

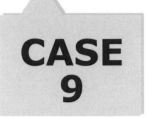

CASE 9

Incisional hernia

Examine this man's abdomen for an incisional hernia.

Incisional hernias occur through an acquired scar in the ventral abdominal wall. Scar tissue is inelastic and never regains its full pre-operative strength. The development of incisional hernias is more likely in wounds which have had infections (up to 10%) or in those which have previously dehisced and were then re-closed (up to 30%).

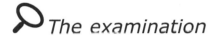

The examination

There will be an abdominal scar. Unless the hernia is large, it may not be immediately obvious with the patient supine. Perform Fothergill's test or ask the patient to cough, and the mass should become obvious in the region of the scar. The raised intra-abdominal pressure will accentuate the hernia and make it easy to define its borders.

Palpation will reveal a defect in the incision and the size will vary. Bowel sounds will often be audible within the defect. Offer to examine the rest of the abdomen.

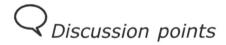

Discussion points

The factors which predispose to incisional hernia formation are summarised below.

Patient factors

- Obesity
- Advanced age
- Impaired tissue healing (diabetes mellitus, steroid use)
- Raised intra-abdominal pressure.

CASE 9

Gastrointestinal disorders

Peri-operative factors

- Infection
- Inadequate closure
- Suture failure
- Haematoma formation
- Post-operative complications – respiratory tract infections.

Many of these hernias, even large ones, can be managed non-surgically with corsets and modification of risk factors (eg weight loss). The risk of strangulation is usually low. Many of these patients are poor operative candidates due to comorbid cardiac or respiratory illnesses.

Most surgeons now advocate the use of polypropylene mesh when surgery is considered, and drain insertion if the defect is large.

CASE
9

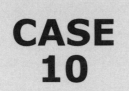

CASE 10

Epigastric mass

Examine this man's abdomen.

The commonest causes of an epigastric mass are carcinoma of the stomach and pancreatic masses (either pseudocysts or carcinomas). However, it is important to note that most gastric carcinomas and pancreatic masses are impalpable. Bearing this in mind, examine the abdomen systematically as you were shown in Case 1.

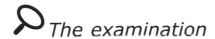 *The examination*

Begin with inspection of the abdomen, followed by light and deep palpation. Inspection may reveal an abnormal contour in the area or scars from previous surgery. When you find the mass, describe it as you would for any lump. Note the site, size, shape, edge, consistency, relationship to surrounding structures, presence of a cough impulse, and whether it is pulsatile and expansile.

Exclude normal causes, such as a prominent left lobe of liver or a nodule in a cirrhotic liver. The best way to construct a differential diagnosis is to understand the structures that are under your hand while you are palpating the epigastrium. These are soft tissues (sarcomas, lipomas or hernias), the liver (cirrhotic nodule or left lobe), the stomach (gastric cancer), the pancreas (pseudocyst or pancreatic carcinoma) and aortic aneurysms.

Complete your examination by looking for peripheral signs which would support your diagnosis, such as anaemia, cachexia, jaundice or lymphadenopathy in the supraclavicular fossa from gastric carcinoma – Troisier's sign (this node is called Virchow's node).

UHB TRUST LIBRARY QEHB

Q *Discussion points*

The features of a mass due to gastric carcinoma are as follows:

- hard, irregular mass
- cannot get above it, extends under costal margin
- moves with respiration.

The features of a mass due to pancreatic pseudocyst are as follows:

- cannot get above it
- poorly defined lower border
- resonant to percussion (air/fluid)
- moves slightly with respiration.

In an OSCE exam, it is more common to be presented with a pseudocyst than with a gastric carcinoma.

**CASE
10**

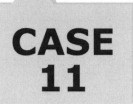

CASE 11

Right iliac fossa mass

Examine this man's abdomen.

This is a common clinical scenario both in exams and in surgical practice. If you are directed to examine the abdomen, proceed as you have already been shown in Case 1. If you are directed to examine the patient first before focusing on the abdomen, start with the hands. The most common causes of a right iliac fossa mass are carcinoma of the caecum, Crohn's disease and an appendix mass. A transplanted third kidney or an ovarian mass are less common causes which arise disproportionately often in exams. Rarely, an ectopic or incompletely descended testis can present in the right iliac fossa, but these cases are unlikely to be available for an OSCE exam.

✐ *The examination*

In Crohn's disease there may also be digital clubbing and anaemia, if the disease is active. Caecal carcinoma often presents insidiously with bleeding, and a mass is only evident in the late stages.

On inspection, there may be asymmetry of the iliac fossae and there may be obvious scars due to previous surgery (renal transplant or laparotomy scars for previous terminal ileal resections in Crohn's disease).

Palpate as before and, depending on the associated features, make your diagnosis.

Q *Discussion points*

Caecal carcinoma – characteristics likely to support the diagnosis

- Elderly patient
- Cachexia may or may not be present
- Anaemia may or may not be present
- Mass is hard and well demarcated
- May be mobile or fixed to abdominal wall
- Non-tender.

Crohn's mass – characteristics likely to support the diagnosis

- Younger patients
- Mobile mass
- Firm consistency, but not hard
- Multiple scars or enterocutaneous fistulae may or may not be present.

The investigation of choice is a contrast CT scan, or an ultrasound scan if ovarian or bladder pathology is suspected.

CASE 11

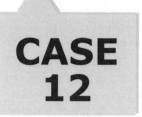

Inflammatory bowel disease and surgery

This woman has inflammatory bowel disease. What are the common operations that are used to treat this condition?

In ulcerative colitis, because there is no involvement of the small bowel the options for surgery are more attractive than for Crohn's disease. Ulcerative colitis starts in the rectum and then spreads proximally, the most common presenting symptom being bloody diarrhoea in an otherwise well patient. If medical treatment with steroids, 5-ASA compounds and immunosuppressants has failed, surgery is indicated.

About one-third of all patients with extensive colitis will require surgery, and about 2% of those with distal disease will require surgery. The acute indications are severe acute colitis, with > 20 bloody motions per day and systemic illness. Perforation or colonic dilatation (megacolon) are absolute indications for intervention, as is massive colorectal bleeding. The more common indication is chronic disease that responds poorly or only partially to medical treatment.

In patients with longstanding ulcerative colitis, of more than 10 years' duration, there is an appreciable risk of malignant transformation.

♀ The examination

In a data station you may be asked for indications for surgery and the types of surgery available. You may be shown an X-ray with megacolon or pneumoperitoneum, or a vital signs chart and a scenario consistent with one of these presentations.

Types of surgery

Historically, complete proctocolectomy was considered the best operation for patients with ulcerative colitis. The entire colon and rectum are removed and a (lifelong) end ileostomy is fashioned. The advantage of this is that the risk of cancer is eliminated and all of the diseased bowel is removed. Unfortunately, the patient is left with a permanent end ileostomy, and around 10% of patients may require stoma revision.

Total colectomy (in which the rectum remains in place) with an ileorectal anastomosis leaves the rectum behind, and with it the inherent risk of disease recurrence or malignant transformation. This procedure is probably only suitable for patients with rectal sparing and those with conditions which would make a rectal dissection dangerous (eg portal hypertension, sclerosing cholangitis).

This situation prevailed until the advent of the restorative proctocolectomy, which is now the operation of choice for most patients, allowing for continence and removal of all diseased bowel. The colon and rectum are removed and the ileum is used to fashion a neorectum (either a J- or a W-pouch). This is then anastomosed to the anal verge – the ileal pouch anal anastomosis (IPAA). Most surgeons defunction the anatomosis with a loop ileostomy higher up, which is then reversed at a later stage. In general, patients prefer the pouch to a permanent ileostomy.

CASE
12

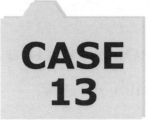

CASE 13

Ulcerative colitis and complications

This young man has ulcerative colitis. What are the complications?

Core knowledge

- Initial symptoms are commonly of diarrhoea, often with bleeding per rectum.
- More severe attacks may be associated with increased frequency of diarrhoea, blood loss causing anaemia, abdominal pain and pyrexia. Increasing severity of symptoms raises the possibility of **toxic megacolon**, which requires emergency surgery.

Discussion points

- The rectosigmoid site is most commonly affected.
- Infective causes of diarrhoea should be excluded.
- Medical treatment may employ steroids, non-steroidal anti-inflammatory compounds and immunomodulatory agents (eg azathioprine, cyclosporin).
- Colectomy is curative in cases that are refractory to medical treatment.
- Complications may be systemic (eg arthritis, iritis, erythema nodosum, sclerosing cholangitis).
- Local complications may include toxic megacolon, perforation, stricture formation, haemorrhage or, in chronic severe disease, malignant transformation.

Advanced issues

- Emergency surgery is indicated when medical therapy has failed or if complications such as megacolon or perforation occur.
- Ileo-anal pouch formation is a means of restoring continuity of the gastrointestinal tract after total colectomy.

CASE 13

CASE 14

Enterocutaneous fistula

What is the abnormality on this woman's abdomen?

This may be presented as a photographic data station or a patient with a fistulous opening on to the skin. Enterocutaneous fistulae are connections between the skin and the bowel, usually the small bowel, which leak enteric contents on to the skin. The commonest cause of these fistulae is abdominal surgery (due to anastomotic leakage, or compromised bowel wall or blood supply), followed by Crohn's disease and penetrating trauma.

⌕ The examination

Patients with fistulae often appear malnourished, dehydrated, or both. On inspection, there may be generalised features of cachexia or extra-intestinal manifestations of Crohn's disease. Often the fistulae will be multiple. The discharge will be enteric and may be copious enough to justify placement of a stoma bag to contain secretions. The examiner will lead a discussion of the aetiology of the fistula.

⌕ Discussion points

In a patient with an enterocutaneous fistula, nutritional and biochemical assessment should include haemoglobin and serum albumin concentrations, body weight and liver function tests. Barium contrast studies are most appropriate for demonstrating areas of small bowel disease, fistulae and even abscesses. Fistulography can provide important information about the complexity of a tract.

Enterocutaneous fistulae usually arise at the site of an anastomosis, or in a segment of non-involved bowel which has been inadvertently damaged during surgery. They are difficult to manage.

Basic management includes correction of fluid and electrolyte imbalance, skin protection and initiation of parenteral intravenous nutrition (see Case 19). Some high-output fistulae can be controlled with the use of somatostatin therapy (octreotide). The fistula anatomy can be defined by contrast imaging. If there is an accompanying abscess, it should be drained.

Around 60–70% of post-anastomotic fistulae heal spontaneously after a period of conservative management, but spontaneous enterocutaneous fistulae rarely heal. These cases usually require surgery to take down the fistula and exteriorise one or both ends as stoma. A new alternative for the treatment of difficult fistulae is anti-TNF-alpha therapy.

Gastrointestinal disorders

CASE 14

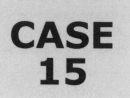

CASE 15

Dysphagia

This man is having difficulty swallowing. Take his history.

Dysphagia is difficulty in swallowing, and odynophagia is painful swallowing. The process of normal swallowing requires co-ordination of complex neural and pharyngeal elements. Dysphagia can result from dysfunction in any of the three phases of swallowing, namely the oral, pharyngeal and oesophageal phases. Aspiration of food contents is a common sequela of dysphagia.

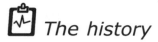

The history

The history is a crucial element of evaluation of the patient with dysphagia. It is important to distinguish it at the outset from odynophagia (painful swallowing associated with infection and neoplasia). You need to ask the patient the following questions.

- Do you have difficulty swallowing liquids, solids, or both?
- Did this problem occur suddenly or gradually?
- Is it getting worse?
- How long is it present for?
- Is it constant or just intermittent?
- Do you vomit immediately?
- Do you regurgitate the food back up?
- Do you eat full meals?
- Are your appetite and weight normal?
- Is it painful to swallow?
- Where do you think the food lodges?

Patients with major oesophageal obstruction commonly regurgitate the bolus after a short period of time. The presence of otalgia can indicate a hypopharyngeal lesion. Any change in diet or weight can indicate the extent of the problem. Neurological problems such as diplopia, dysarthria and altered mental status can indicate a central nervous system aetiology. In patients with intermittent dysphagia, the cause may be dysmotility or supratentorial.

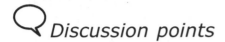 *Discussion points*

Causes of dysphagia

- Neurological causes – cerebrovascular accident, trauma, multiple sclerosis, amyotrophic lateral sclerosis, cerebral palsy, motor neurone disease/bulbar palsy
- Muscular causes – connective tissue disease, oropharyngeal muscular dystrophy
- Motility – achalasia, Zenker's diverticulum
- Obstruction – oesophageal carcinoma, strictures, webs, rings.

Factors which contribute to dysphagia

- Hyposalivation (eg due to radiation therapy), which makes it difficult to initiate the swallow
- Insertion of a tracheostomy tube (see Case 28), which limits laryngeal elevation

Oesophageal carcinoma usually presents with gradually worsening dysphagia, first for solids and then for liquids, with associated weight loss. Often there is associated odynophagia. The use of dilators or stenting will relieve obstruction, and treatment consists of pre-operative chemoradiotherapy followed by oesophagectomy in patients who have localised disease. Palliative treatment will allow resumption of swallowing.

The investigations of choice for all structural or motility causes are endoscopy and biopsy, with barium swallow to diagnose motility problems such as oesophageal spasm or achalasia.

Gastrointestinal disorders

CASE 15

CASE 16

Peptic ulcer disease

A 35-year-old man with a history of duodenal ulcer presents to you with upper abdominal pain that has been present for 4 days. It has now become much worse and is associated with vomiting and back pain.

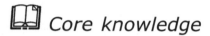 *Core knowledge*

Differential diagnosis

- Duodenal/gastric ulceration
- Perforated viscus
- Gastritis
- Biliary disease
- Pancreatitis.

Essential investigations

- Gastroscopy
- Campylobacter like organism (CLO) test
- Ultrasound examination of abdomen.

Discussion points

- *Helicobacter pylori* and its management (eradicate with triple therapy consisting of a proton-pump inhibitor and two antibiotics)
- Complications of excess alcohol ingestion
- The differential management of duodenal and gastric ulceration (gastric ulcers must be biopsied to exclude malignancy). The treatment is now primarily medical, with surgery being reserved for refractory cases or those who develop complications such as perforation or bleeding.

CASE
16

🎓 *Advanced knowledge*

- The surgical treatment of perforated duodenal ulcer should include oversewing with an omental patch.
- Biopsy method for gastric ulcers (four-quadrant technique, with double biopsy).

Gastrointestinal disorders

CASE 16

CASE 17

Clubbing

Examine this man's hands and tell me what you think.

Digital clubbing was first described in patients with empyema by Hippocrates. It is an increase in the amount of soft tissue at the distal end of the fingers and toes.

Clubbing is a sign of underlying pulmonary, cardiovascular, gastrointestinal, neoplastic or endocrine disease. It can also occur in the absence of any underlying disease, in an idiopathic form or as a Mendelian dominant trait. It can arise with equal frequency in medical and surgical OSCE stations.

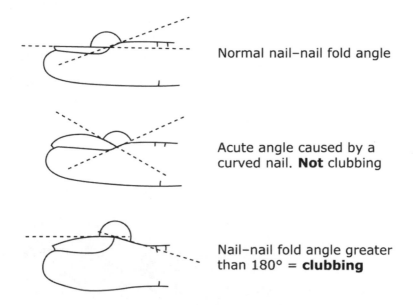

Normal nail–nail fold angle

Acute angle caused by a curved nail. **Not** clubbing

Nail–nail fold angle greater than 180° = **clubbing**

Fig 4 Demonstration of loss of the nail bed angle in clubbing

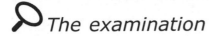 *The examination*

The case will be obvious. Although clubbing can be limited to a single digit, these cases will not be brought for exams. As always, direct the patient courteously and expose their hands and arms up to the elbows. Always allow the patient to move their hands rather than you, to avoid causing them pain.

On inspection, it will be obvious whether or not clubbing is present. Kneel and inspect the anteroposterior curvature of the nails. In clubbing this is greater than 180º. Is there loss of angle between the nail and the nailbed? Compare the patient's finger with your own, and also with the same finger on their opposite hand. In a person with normal digits there will be a diamond shape between the two nailbeds – the 'diamond' sign or Lovibond's sign. 'Drumsticking' of the terminal phalanges is a late sign.

Palpation will reveal bogginess of the nailbed, making it easy for you to rock it from side to side after you have asked the patient if they have any pain. Test each digit in turn, using your thumbs to support the digit and your index fingers to test for fluctuance.

Complete your examination by asking to examine the toes, palpating the wrists for joint tenderness (hypertrophic pulmonary osteoarthropathy, HPOA), and asking about symptoms which could be referable to any of the causes listed below.

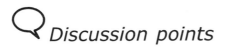 *Discussion points*

HPOA is associated with primary lung carcinoma and mesothelioma. It is caused by periosteal inflammation at the end of long bones (the wrists, ankles, etc). Rarely, HPOA may occur without clubbing.

When clubbing develops suddenly and is painful, one should suspect bronchogenic carcinoma.

**CASE
17**

The causes of clubbing are listed below (asterisks indicate the most common causes).

- Idiopathic – most common cause*
- Cardiovascular causes

    Cyanotic congenital heart disease*

    Infective endocarditis
- Pulmonary causes

    Lung carcinoma* (but not small-cell carcinoma)

    Any suppurative lung process

      Empyema*

      Bronchiectasis*

    Cystic fibrosis

    Mesothelioma
- Gastrointestinal causes

    Inflammatory bowel disease

    Coeliac disease

    Cirrhosis
- Endocrine causes

    Thyrotoxicosis.

The exact pathophysiology of clubbing is not known, but many studies have shown that there is an increase in distal digital vasodilatation. As yet it is unclear whether this is due to the action of a local or circulating vasodilator, a neural mechanism, or a response to hypoxaemia.

Support for the theory that a circulating vasodilator is the cause comes from the association with congenital cyanotic heart disease. There are many potential vasodilators, which are usually inactivated when blood is filtered through the lungs. However, they bypass this inactivation process when there is a right-to-left shunt. Clubbing is particularly severe in patients with tetralogy of Fallot, and improves with correction of the shunt.

**CASE
17**

CASE 18

Enteral feeding

This cachetic patient with oesophageal cancer requires supplemental nutrition.

 Core knowledge

- Malnutrition is very common in patients with malignant disease. This may be due to tumour-specific problems such as dysphagia, or secondary to the hypermetabolic state that is seen with some tumours.

- Malnutrition places patients at increased risk of post-operative complications, including wound healing and repair, which may cause problems with incision and anastomosis healing.

- Feeding during the peri-operative period is very important in order to reduce operation-specific and infection-related complications.

 Discussion points

- Enteral feeding has advantages over parenteral feeding in terms of the following:

    (i)   Central venous access lines are unnecessary, so their technical and infective complications are avoided.

    (ii)   Enteral feeding may aid immunological function, with preservation of the gut mucosal barrier.

- Subjective global assessment of malnutrition and calorie requirements.

Advanced issues

- Oesophageal dilation with or without stenting may allow oral feeding to recommence.
- Multimodality treatment is becoming more widespread, and nutritional support is necessary during this time.

CASE
18

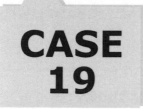

CASE 19

Parenteral nutrition

You are shown a post-operative patient on parenteral nutrition.

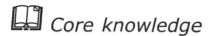 *Core knowledge*

Complications of total parenteral nutrition include the following:

- infective complications – line sepsis
- metabolic complications – hyperosmolar states, liver function abnormalities, hyperglycaemia
- technical complications – haemopneumothorax/pneumothorax from line insertion.

Normal calorie requirements are 2500 kcal/day.

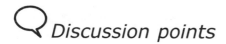 *Discussion points*

- The need for vitamin and mineral support with total parenteral nutrition.
- Factors that increase caloric requirements: burns, sepsis, trauma and any catabolic state.

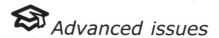 *Advanced issues*

Role and indications for total parenteral nutrition at home (eg short bowel syndrome).

CASE 19

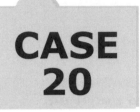

CASE 20

Large bowel obstruction

What does this X-ray show?

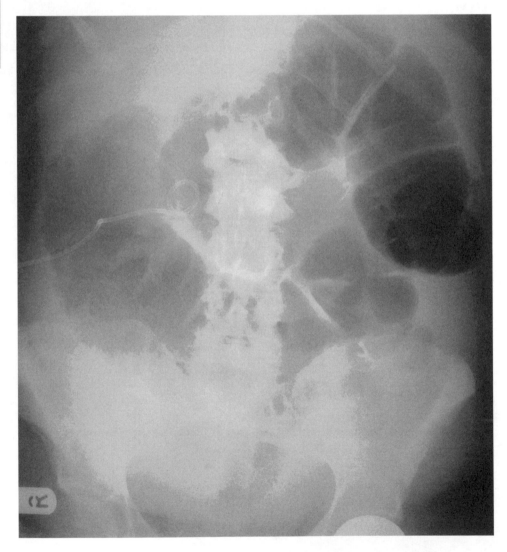

Fig 5 Plain film of the abdomen showing large bowel obstruction

CASE
20

Core knowledge

- Obstruction may be caused by an obstructing lesion (malignant or benign stricture), adhesions, volvulus or herniation, or there may be no identifiable cause, as in pseudo-obstruction.
- Crampy pain, distension, absolute constipation and vomiting are the cardinal symptoms of obstruction.

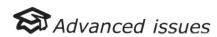 # Discussion points

- Large bowel obstruction is an urgent surgical condition which, if left untreated, may result in caecal perforation.
- Immediate management consists of fluid and electrolyte replacement with nasogastric drainage, in parallel with investigations to determine the cause.

 # Advanced issues

- Pseudo-obstruction must be ruled out before surgery.
- Surgical options may include a Hartman's procedure or on-table lavage and primary anastomosis.

**CASE
20**

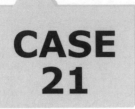

Gastrointestinal disorders

CASE 21

Data – faecal occult blood (FOB) test/sigmoidoscopy

What is this used for?

 Core knowledge

- Faecal occult blood positivity may lead to a sigmoidoscopy or a colonoscopy.
- Flexible sigmoidoscopy can detect up to 70% of colon cancers.

Discussion points

- Sigmoidoscopy must be complemented by either barium enema or colonoscopy for complete colonic assessment.
- FOB tests may be associated with upper gastrointestinal blood loss, as well as with false-positive readings.

Advanced issues

- Right-sided colonic tumours are less likely to present with obstructive symptoms than left-sided tumours.
- Genetic screening for the adenomatous polyposis coli (APC) gene is a useful test for family members in cases where familial polyposis coli is suspected.

CASE 22

Data – CLO test for *Helicobacter pylori*

What is this?

 ## Core knowledge

- *Helicobacter pylori* is a risk factor for diseases such as peptic ulceration, duodenitis and gastritis.
- The organism can be eradicated by antibiotic treatment.

Discussion points

- *H. pylori* Is a recognised carcinogen associated with gastric cancer.
- The campylobacter like organism (CLO) test relies on the urease activity of *H. pylori*.

 ## Advanced issues

- Breath testing, immunoglobulin serology and microscopy are other methods of testing for *H. pylori*.
- *H. pylori* induces mucosal damage by production of urease and ammonia, acetaldehyde and mucolytic factors, as well as having a chemotactic effect on polymorphs.

Gastrointestinal disorders

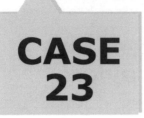

CASE 23

Data – full blood count with anaemia

The full blood count shows hypochromic microcytic anaemia.

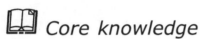

Core knowledge

Hypochromic microcytic anaemia represents iron-deficiency anaemia that is most commonly associated with gastrointestinal loss. Other causes include thalassaemia and anaemia of chronic dieases.

Causes of gastrointestinal blood loss include the following:

- upper gastrointestinal ulceration, inflammation, or tumour of the oesophagus, stomach or duodenum
- lower gastrointestinal diverticulosis, carcinoma, polyp, inflammatory bowel disease or angiodysplasia
- miscellaneous causes, including aorto-enteric fistula, small bowel angiodysplasia or Meckel's diverticulum.

Discussion points

- In the patient's history, use of prescribed or over-the-counter non-steroidal anti-inflammatory medications should be sought, as well as anticoagulant or steroid usage.
- Initial investigations will be guided by symptoms, and may include faecal occult blood testing and iron, vitamin B_{12} and folate levels.
- Endoscopy of the upper and lower gastrointestinal tracts is usually performed, and complete visualisation by endoscopic or radiological methods is mandatory if the cause of anaemia is unclear.

Advanced issues

- If endoscopy fails to identify a bleeding source, angiography and labelled red-cell scans may be used, although they will only identify active bleeding points.
- Small bowel bleeding may be identified by capsule endoscopy, usually as a second-line investigation for recurrent episodes.

Gastrointestinal disorders

CASE
23

Gastrointestinal disorders

CASE 24

Barium enema with diverticular disease

What does this X-ray show?

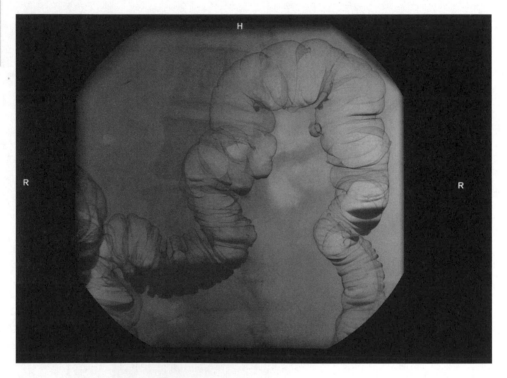

Fig 6 Barium enema showing diverticulae

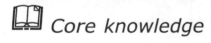 Core knowledge

- Diverticular disease is predominantly located on the left side of the colon, and is extremely common in the western world.

- Presentation may include pain, altered bowel habit, bleeding per rectum or, in an acute setting, left iliac pain and tenderness associated with pyrexia and leukocytosis in acute diverticulitis.

CASE
24

Discussion point

Complications of diverticular disease may include the following:

- acute infection – diverticulitis
- bleeding
- stricture formation
- fistulation
- perforation.

The management of acute diverticulitis includes intravenous antibiotics and observation. CT scanning may be employed to detect pericolic abscess formation, which can then be drained percutaneously.

Surgery is indicated for acute perforation, intractable haemorrhage or fistulation.

Advanced issues

- Careful investigation is necessary, as carcinoma may coexist with diverticular disease.
- Colonoscopy should be attempted with care, as perforation is possible if the scope passes into a diverticulum.

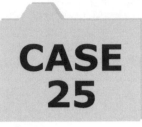

Gastrointestinal disorders

CASE 25

Pneumoperitoneum

What does this X-ray show?

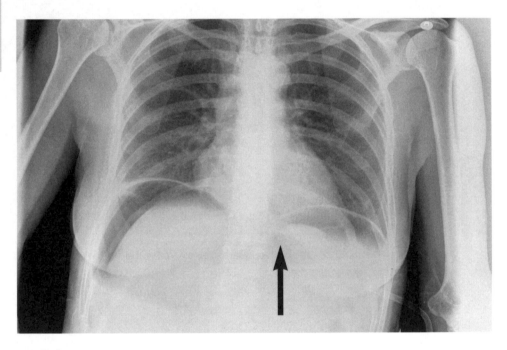

Fig 7 Free air under the diaphragm

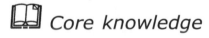

📖 Core knowledge

- Free air under the diaphragm is highly suggestive of visceral perforation.
- The absence of free air does not exclude perforation (40% of cases).

CASE
25

ℚ Discussion points

- Erect chest X-ray is the appropriate investigation for detecting free air.
- The commonest causes are perforated peptic ulceration and perforated diverticular disease.

🎓 Advanced issues

- Primary bacterial peritonitis may give an appearance of free air.
- Free air may persist for several days after laparotomy or laparoscopy.
- Peptic ulcer perforation may on occasion be treated conservatively with fluid resuscitation, antibiotics and nasogastric aspiration. Standard treatment includes surgical closure of the perforation.

CASE 25

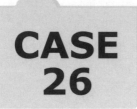

CASE 26

Gastrointestinal bleeding

You are in the Emergency department when a 60-year-old man is brought in following an episode of haematemesis. What are the initial measures which should be taken and what are the likely causes in this man?

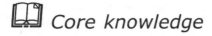 *Core knowledge*

The use of role-play scenarios in OSCE exams is becoming more common, and you will be expected to be competent in the management of a number of emergency situations. Upper gastrointestinal haemorrhage occurs proximal to the ligament of Treitz and is characterised by haematemesis and later by the passage of melaena. If there is massive haemorrhage, the blood may pass unaltered via the rectum – this is termed haematochezia.

The commonest causes of upper gastrointestinal haemorrhage demonstrated at endoscopy are as follows:

- duodenal ulcer (40% of cases)
- gastric ulcer (10–20%)
- erosive gastritis (15–20%)
- oesophageal varices (10%)
- Mallory–Weiss tear of the gastro-oesophageal junction (10%)
- gastric carcinoma (< 5%).

This is a life-threatening emergency, and although the diagnosis of acute haemorrhage is often obvious, location of the site of the bleeding can be difficult. The immediate measure which should be taken is placement of wide-bore peripheral cannulae or a central venous catheter if access is difficult. This should be followed immediately by infusion of an adequate amount of colloid to maintain intravascular volume. Blood for estimation of full blood count and clotting status as well as for crossmatching should be taken now. The history should include the use of any anticoagulant medications (aspirin and warfarin are common), previous episodes of gastrointestinal bleeding and any related systemic diseases (eg alcoholism, peptic ulcer disease, haematological disorders, recent episodes of forceful vomiting).

The physical examination must specifically search for evidence of portal hypertension, malignancy, nasopharyngeal bleeding and systemic diseases such as hepatic or renal failure.

The goal of resuscitation is to arrest haemorrhage and maintain blood flow to vital organs. Only when this has been achieved should diagnostic tests be considered.

Checklist for management of gastrointestinal haemorrhage

✓ Use the ABC approach, ensure airway, breathing and circulation in that order

✓ Wide-bore cannulae or central venous catheter.

✓ Rapid infusion of colloid to correct hypotension.

✓ Estimation of haemoglobin and clotting status, and blood for crossmatching.

✓ Monitoring of blood pressure, pulse, oxygen saturations and hourly urine output.

✓ Pass a nasogastric tube to decompress the stomach and reduce the risk of aspiration.

✓ Commence infusion of proton-pump inhibitors or antacids. H2-receptor antagonists are ineffective in stopping haemorrhage.

✓ Give fresh frozen plasma if the prothrombin time is abnormal, and give platelets if thrombocytopaenia is present.

✓ Give blood when available if blood pressure is not maintained by clear fluids.

✓ Give unmatched blood O-negative if necessary if the haemorrhage is massive.

✓ Correct coagulopathies.

✓ Intervene early in cases with chronic disease or atherosclerosis, as these patients do not tolerate hypotension well.

✓ Fibre-optic endoscopy is the intervention of choice in patients who stabilise following resuscitation.

CASE 26

Q *Discussion points*

Most patients with upper gastrointestinal haemorrhage make an excellent recovery. In your exam, you must convey the fact that resuscitation takes priority over diagnosis, and outline the core principles of resuscitation as shown above.

When haemorrhage is due to oesophageal varices, the use of a Sengstaken–Blakemore tube to tamponade the variceal vessels is indicated. Vasopressin (a potent vasoconstrictor) can be used to control bleeding, and is effective in 75% of patients. It reduces cardiac output, and is contraindicated in coronary artery disease.

The indications for surgery are as follows:

- exsanguinating haemorrhage, where blood is being lost faster than it can be replaced
- profuse bleeding, especially if it is associated with hypotension. Treat surgically if more than four units of blood are required for the initial resuscitation, if there is an ongoing transfusion requirement of more than one unit every 8 hours, or if hypotension could have catastrophic results (eg in patients over 60 years of age, and in those with coronary artery or cerebrovascular disease)
- continued haemorrhage despite resuscitation and treatment
- recurrent bleeding after cessation. About 25% of patients rebleed, and this group may have a mortality rate of up to 30%.

**CASE
26**

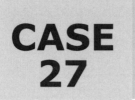

CASE 27

Left iliac fossa pain

This woman has a 10-day history of left iliac fossa pain. How would you manage her problem?

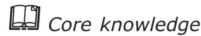

Core knowledge

In an elderly woman, the likely diagnosis is diverticular disease. In a younger patient, you should consider gynaecological causes such as an ovarian cyst. Enquire about any changes in bowel habit that might suggest diverticular disease. Bleeding per rectum could be due to diverticular disease, but could also be associated with carcinoma of the colon. In a younger patient, it is important to ascertain the relationship between pain and the menstrual cycle.

If acute diverticular disease is diagnosed, management should include nil by mouth, intravenous fluids and intravenous antibiotics. The chosen antibiotics should include an agent that is effective against anaerobic organisms, such as metronidazole. A CT scan is useful for assessing the complications of diverticular disease, such as abscess formation or perforation. If an abscess has developed, radiological drainage can usually be performed. If a perforation has occurred, surgical intervention is required. This usually necessitates a Hartman's procedure, in which the diseased section of bowel is resected, the proximal end is brought out as a stoma and the distal end is oversewn.

Discussion points

- How might diverticular disease be avoided? Discuss the issues in relation to a high-fibre diet.
- Is it necessary to evaluate the inside of the bowel in diverticular disease? To avoid missing a colorectal carcinoma, the inside of the bowel should be evaluated either at colonoscopy or by means of a barium enema before making a definitive diagnosis that excludes colorectal carcinoma.
- How might an ovarian cyst be diagnosed? In young female patients, ultrasound examination is particularly valuable. You may see the cyst, or if it has ruptured you may see free fluid in the pouch of Douglas.

CASE 27

Thoracic disorders

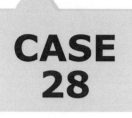

CASE 28

Tracheostomy

What is this device?

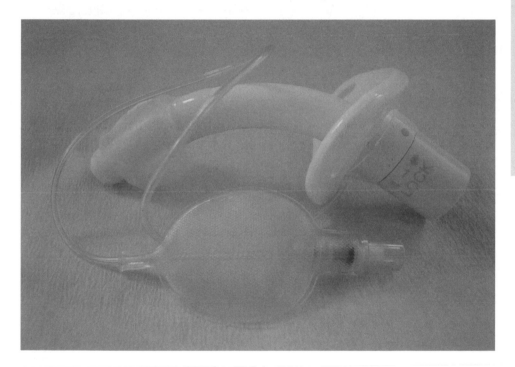

Fig 8 Tracheostomy tube

This is a tracheostomy tube. A tracheostomy is a surgical procedure for creating an artificial opening or **stoma** into the trachea. It may be temporary or permanent, and it runs from the second to the fourth tracheal ring. There are many different types of tracheostomy tube, one of which is shown here. These devices are often available to exam supervisors, and are a source of much confusion among students.

There are many reasons for performing a tracheostomy. In surgical patients, they are most often placed in the presence of severe maxillofacial injury, in patients who require a prolonged period (> 2 weeks) of oral or nasal endotracheal intubation, or in those who have had laryngectomy performed because of malignancy.

Thoracic disorders

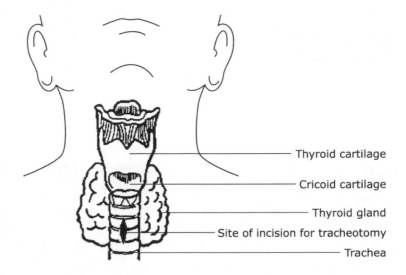

Fig 9 Anatomy at the site of a tracheostomy

Medical indications for tracheostomy include the following:

- airway problems (eg vocal cord paralysis)
- sleep apnoea
- congenital abnormalities (eg Treacher Collins' syndrome, Pierre Robin's syndrome)
- lung problems (eg chronic pulmonary disease) to reduce dead space.

The procedure can be performed in theatre under general anaesthesia or in the ICU by a guidewire technique, via the percutaneous tract.

In the exam you may also be asked about complications of tracheostomy insertion. These include the following:

- respiratory distress due to tube obstruction
- bleeding
- infection (loss of mucociliary defences)
- tracheal stenosis
- tracheoesophageal fistula.

CASE
28

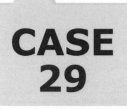

CASE 29

Pneumothorax

What does this X-ray show?

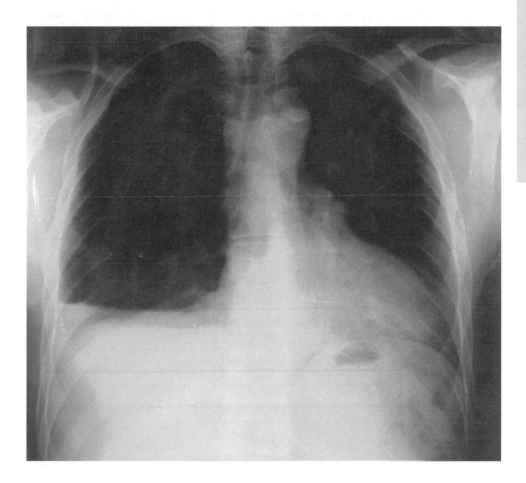

Fig 10 OXR demonstrating a pneumothorax

Core knowledge

This is air in the pleural space. It may occur spontaneously or after trauma. The air may enter through a chest wound or as a result of damage to the trachea, oesophagus or main bronchus. In most cases the leak is from the lung itself. In hospital, it can occur following central venous cannulation, during intermittent positive pressure ventilation or even during a prolonged asthmatic attack.

Spontaneous pneumothoraces can be due to localised lung disease (focal, air-filled cysts or solitary bullae, often in tall young men) or generalised lung disease (usually in elderly smokers with severe bullous emphysema or other fibrosing lung conditions).

Discussion points

- Management of pneumothorax is not initially influenced by its aetiology. Small pneumothoraces can be observed if the patient is asymptomatic and the air is being resorbed on serial chest X-ray. Larger ones require chest-tube insertion.

- Tension pneumothorax is an emergency. Its treatment is described elsewhere in this section (see Case 30).

Advanced knowledge

Surgery for recurrent or troublesome pneumothorax (ie open pleurectomy or video-assisted thorascopic surgery with control of the air leak).

CASE 29

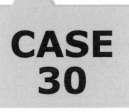

CASE 30

Chest drain

What is this medical device?

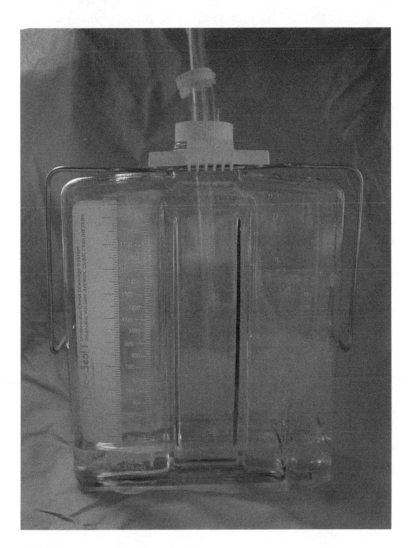

Fig 11 An underwater seal

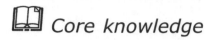 *Core knowledge*

- Chest drains are used for the treatment of pneumothoraces, haemothoraces and pleural effusions, and following thoracic trauma or surgery.

- An underwater seal is used as a one-way valve when chest drains are used to treat pneumothoraces.

- Chest drains should be inserted in the fifth intercostal space in the mid-axillary line or in the second intercostal space in the mid-clavicular line.

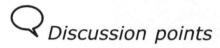 *Discussion points*

- Clinical findings in pneumothorax (absent breath sounds, hyper-resonant to percussion on affected side).

- The management of a tension pneumothorax. It is important to perform a needle thoracostomy if this is clinically suspected (absent breath sounds, respiratory distress, tracheal shift away from affected side). Take a chest X-ray prior to chest drain placement.

- An expiratory film demonstrates pneumothoraces best, as the underlying lung becomes denser, making the air trapped in the pleural space easier to see.

Advanced knowledge

- Recurrent spontaneous pneumothorax is treated by pleurodesis, either through open surgery or by video-assisted thorascopic surgery.

- The complications of chest drain insertion include haemorrhage, cardiac or splenic injury on the left, and liver injury on the right. When the procedure is used to drain pleural effusions, the fluid should be removed slowly to minimise re-expansion pulmonary oedema).

Thoracic disorders

**CASE
30**

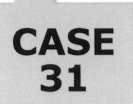

CASE 31

Sternotomy/ thoracotomy

Examine this man's chest (patient with sternotomy/thoracotomy scar).

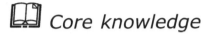 *Core knowledge*

- Sternotomy leaves a central scar from the suprasternal notch to the epigastrium. This is used to access the mediastinal structures and the heart in open cardiac procedures (for congenital abnormalities in children or for coronary artery surgery in adults).

- Sternotomy incision may also be used to access a retrosternal thyroid goitre or the thoracic aorta. The presence of a sternotomy scar may prompt a discussion about coronary artery disease and arteriopathy in general.

- Thoracotomy incisions are commonly used to access the lung for the purpose of lobectomy either in cases of malignancy or for bullous disease.

Discussion points

The complications of the above incisions include herniation (sternotomy) and neuralgia (thoracotomy).

General

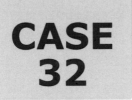

CASE 32

Splenomegaly

Examine this young man's abdomen.

Splenomegaly has many causes, and they are best classified according to the underlying pathological process. There are not many extra-abdominal signs in patients with splenomegaly who are brought for exams, but you may see peripheral evidence of anaemia or rheumatoid arthritis. The spleen is part of the reticulo-endothelial system, and its main functions are to sequester the old blood cells from the circulation, to produce IgM and filter out pathogens, and to store platelets.

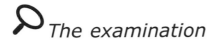

The examination

Position, expose and direct the patient as described for the abdominal examination. Usually the spleen enlarges uniformly, and it may give a visible impression of fullness under the left costal margin when there is massive splenomegaly. More commonly, there will be no abnormalities on inspection.

On palpation, begin in the right iliac fossa as the spleen enlarges diagonally across the mid-line. On inspiration, keep your palpating hand stationary, and with each expiration advance it towards the left hypochondrium. The edge will be felt below the costal margin. If the edge is not felt, place your left hand on the left costal margin and pull the rib-cage forward. Occasionally, the splenic edge will become more obvious. If this fails, roll the patient on to their right side and begin palpation near the left costal margin. You will not have to do this in the exam, but describe the procedure to the examiners if you are asked. This could also be a massively enlarged left kidney, and therefore you must have some means of distinguishing between the alternatives.

Features of an enlarged spleen include the following:

- It appears from below the tip of the left tenth rib and enlarges along the line of the rib towards the umbilicus. It can cross the mid-line.
- You cannot get above it.
- It moves with respiration.
- It may have a notch on the lower border, but this is not always so.
- It cannot be balloted, unlike an enlarged left kidney.

CASE 32

There may be associated hepatomegaly, as seen in chronic liver disease with portal hypertension, some haematological illnesses such as lymphoma, leukaemia and myeloproliferative disease, and also infiltrative processes such as amyloidosis or sarcoidosis.

Q Discussion points

The causes of splenomegaly are listed below. They can be categorised by aetiology or by extent of organomegaly.

Causes according to aetiology

- Infection

    Bacterial (typhoid, typhus, TB)

    Sepsis

    Protozoans (malaria or kala-azar)

    Viral (infectious mononucleosis)

- Infarction

    Emboli from bacterial endocarditis or the left atrium

    Splenic artery or vein thrombosis

- Infiltration

    Amyloidosis

    Gaucher's disease

    Sarcoidosis

- Systemic causes

    Rheumatoid arthritis

- Proliferative causes

    Leukaemias

    Idiopathic thrombocytopenic purpura

    Spherocytosis.

Causes according to size

- Massive

    Myelofibrosis

    Chronic myeloid leukaemia

CASE
32

Primary lymphoma

Kala-azar

Malaria

- Moderate

Portal hypertension

Lymphoma

Acute or chronic leukaemias

Gaucher's disease

All of the above

- Mild

Polycythaemia rubra vera

Haemolytic anaemias

Infective causes

Infiltrative causes (amyloidosis, sarcoidosis)

All of the above.

Massive splenomegaly is not common in the developed world, but you should be aware of the causes. These include malaria, myelofibrosis, myeloid leukaemia (chronic) and visceral leishmaniasis (kala-azar).

The commonest indication for splenectomy is trauma. Although splenic conservation is now practised using mesh bags for repair, most seriously damaged spleens are removed. The other common indications for splenectomy are diseases which cause hypersplenism, such as congenital spherocytosis, autoimmune or thrombotic thrombocytopaenias and (rarely) myelofibrotic disorders.

Post-splenectomy prophylaxis against overwhelming post-splenectomy infection (OPSI) can vary from one region to another. However, it should include vaccination in the post-operative period against pneumococci, *Haemophilus influenzae* and meningococci, with lifelong penicillin prophylaxis and annual vaccination against influenza strains.

General

CASE
32

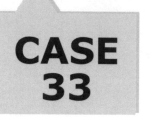

CASE 33

Lump – general approach

You are shown a patient with a soft tissue swelling.

Core knowledge

- Look

    Site, with respect to a bony landmark

    Size (in centimetres)

    Shape (is it regular or not?)

    Scars in the area (is it recurrent?)

    Symmetry

    Colour of the lesion and surrounding area

- Palpate surface texture

    Edge (is demarcation well or poorly defined?)

    Consistency (is it soft or firm/hard?)

    Temperature – use the back of your hand to test this (is it warm or not?)

    Tenderness

    Is it pulsatile or expansile (fingers pushed apart)?

    Is it compressible or reducible?

- Percuss

    Is it dull or resonant?

- Auscultate

    Are there bruits or bowel sounds (possible hernia)?

- Transilluminate

    In a darkened room, using a pen torch from the side, look down an opaque tube.

🎓 Advanced issues

- Always look for similar lumps elsewhere.
- Assess the regional lymph nodes.
- Evaluate the neurovascular integrity of the area.

General

CASE
33

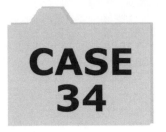

CASE 34

Abdominal scars

Examine the abdomen of this patient.

You will be asked to examine the abdomen of a patient with surgical scars. Remember to introduce yourself, wash your hands, and obtain adequate exposure while maintaining the patient's dignity.

📖 Core knowledge

- The key is to know the descriptive terms for the incision you are presented with, not to attempt to state the operation that it was for.
- At the end of the case, the examiner may ask you to speculate about the nature of the operation involved.
- Remember to look for groin scars and to inspect the back of the patient. You should also check whether there are any scars from previous stoma formation.

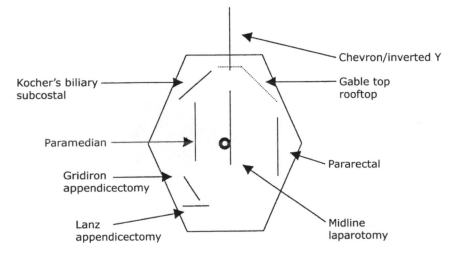

Fig 12 Abdominal incisions

General

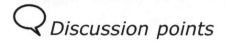 *Discussion points*

After the naming of the particular scar, the topics of wound healing and incisional hernias are favourites of examiners.

General

CASE
34

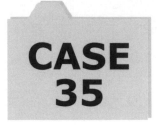

CASE 35

Sebaceous cysts

Examine these swellings.

These are extremely common. You should apply the principles discussed earlier in relation to inspection of any soft tissue swelling.

Core knowledge

- On inspection, these swellings are usually solitary, have a smooth outline and are most commonly found on the face, trunk, neck or scalp.

- On palpation, they are smooth textured, with a variable consistency. They have a punctum, and they do not move independently of the skin, as they are attached to it.

- Complications include infection, ulceration, keratin horn formation and (rarely) malignant change.

Discussion points

- Treatment is non-surgical if the cysts are small and asymptomatic. If they are painful or there is a cosmetic issue, then they may be removed intact with an ellipse of skin to minimise recurrence.

- Sebaceous cysts may sometimes be quite large and resemble a squamous-cell carcinoma. In these circumstances they are known as Cock's peculiar tumours.

🎓 Advanced knowledge

- Sebaceous cysts are also part of Gardner's syndrome, which consists of familial adenomatous polyposis with multiple osteomas of the skull, skin fibromas and epidermoid cysts.
- Histologically, there are two main variants of cysts, namely epidermal cysts, which arise from the infundibular portions of hair follicles, and trichilemmal cysts, which arise from the hair-follicle epithelium.

General

CASE 35

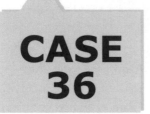

CASE 36

Lipomas

These should be examined as discussed earlier in relation to any soft tissue swelling.

Lipomas are very common and may occur anywhere in the body, but are especially common in the trunk and neck.

 Core knowledge

- Lipomas are benign tumours composed of fat cells. They are discoid or hemispherical swellings which can appear lobulated, and they may recur.
- They are not attached to the overlying skin, and are usually found in the subcutaneous layers.
- In general, they cause problems due to their size or cosmetic issues.
- Treatment of lipomas is by observation if they are asymptomatic, or surgical excision if they are painful, or for cosmetic reasons.

Discussion points

- Liposarcomas are malignant tumours of the deeper tissues which occur in older patients and are probably not related to lipomas.
- In Dercum's disease there are multiple, painful lipomas with an associated peripheral neuropathy.

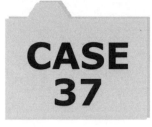

CASE 37

Seborrhoeic keratoses

Examine these lesions.

These are light or dark brown raised papular lesions (also known as senile keratoses), which can be confused with malignant pigmented lesions. Treatment is by excision.

 ## Core knowledge

- These lesions have a 'stuck-on' appearance, and can be picked off to reveal tiny capillaries. The degree of pigmentation is variable, but they may be difficult to distinguish from melanoma in some cases.
- Do not forget to ask about similar lesions elsewhere, and whether the patient would like to have them removed, and if so, why.
- There is an overgrowth of the basal cell layer of the epidermis, characterised by hyperkeratosis, acanthosis and hyperplasia of basaloid cells, which cause the pigmentation.
- Seborrhoeic keratoses may be excised for diagnostic or cosmetic reasons.

Advanced knowledge

The abrupt advent of multiple seborrhoeic keratoses is associated with visceral malignancy. This is called the Leser–Trélat sign.

General

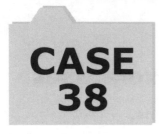

CASE 38

Ganglia

These can occur in areas of weakened retinaculum, leading to outpouching of the underlying synovial structures. Although their origin is uncertain, it seems most likely that they develop as a result of myxomatous degeneration of fibrous tissue. They most commonly occur in areas of the hands and feet that are subjected to repeated minor trauma. Recurrences are common if the ganglion is not excised intact.

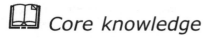 *Core knowledge*

- Ganglia are usually demonstrated in the hands, so after telling the patient what you plan to do, expose their hands and arms. It is courteous to ensure that the ganglion is not painful, and to provide a pillow on which the patient can place their hands.

- They are usually solitary, and there may be a previous scar as they may be recurrent. They are smooth to the touch and may be multiloculated, although this is normally only apparent at operation. Ganglia are usually tense and do not actually communicate with the joint.

- They are almost always associated with a tendon or a joint (ie a synovial lined structure), and they are slow-growing.

- The main differential diagnoses are bursae and cystic protrusions of the synovial cavity in patients with rheumatoid arthritis. Ganglia can be removed by excision under tourniquet control.

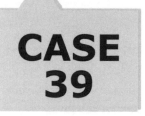

CASE 39

Basal-cell carcinoma and squamous-cell carcinoma

These will be considered together as they often occur on the same exam, and may even be in the same bay.

Basal-cell carcinoma (BCC)

 ## Core knowledge

This is a locally invasive carcinoma which, although it cannot metastasise, can kill by infiltration of local structures. It is the commonest skin cancer, and It usually presents as a slow-growing nodule in a sun-exposed area of the face. The nodule repeatedly falls off and will not heal. If neglected, it can invade local structures and become painful (the so-called 'rodent ulcer').

The main differential diagnosis is squamous-cell carcinoma or a keratoacanthoma with a sloughing centre. In contrast to squamous-cell carcinomas, which have a raised and everted edge, basal-cell carcinomas have a raised and rolled edge with a pearlescent tint due to the fine blood vessels within.

Take care to examine the draining lymph nodes for all skin lesions, which in this case should not be enlarged.

 ## Discussion points

- The different clinical types of basal-cell carcinoma are nodular, cystic, an ulcer proper, a rodent ulcer (fixed to deep structures), a pigmented nodule and the so-called 'forest-fire' type, which has an advancing edge and healing centre.
- The different histological types are superficial, nodular, pigmented (which can be confused with melanoma) and morphea-like (sclerosing).
- Discuss the predisposing factors for skin cancer, namely age, ultraviolet radiation, ionising radiation following adjuvant therapy for other malignancies, and chemical carcinogens.

General

CASE 39

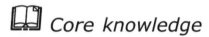Advanced issues

- The treatment options include local excision only with primary closure, and excision with grafting if necessary.
- Basal-cell carcinoma may also be associated with xeroderma pigmentosum, a congenital defect of DNA transcription, or it may be found in unstable burns (Curling's ulcer). BCC may also be found in Gorlin's syndrome, an autosomal-dominant inherited condition characterised by multiple BCCs early in life, mesenteric cysts and scoliosis.

Squamous-cell carcinoma (SCC)

Core knowledge

These skin cancers tend to be quite vascular and often bleed, in contrast to basal-cell carcinoma. When examining these cases, be aware that nodal and distant metastases are common in advanced tumours.

Squamous-cell carcinoma is a carcinoma of the cells of the epidermis, which under normal circumstances migrate outwards to form the superficial keratinous squamous layer. It accounts for about 25% of all skin cancers and is both locally aggressive and capable of metastasis.

Examine as for any lump, but note that SCC has several distinguishing features.

- It has a raised everted edge.
- It is reddish-brown in colour due to vascularity.
- It often has central ulceration.
- It more commonly bleeds than BCC.

The incidence of nodal metastases at presentation is of the order of 5% for SCC. The regions of the body that are most commonly involved are sun-exposed areas, especially the head and neck.

General

**CASE
39**

Q *Discussion points*

- Predisposing factors are xeroderma pigmentosum (as already discussed for BCC), human papillomavirus 5 and 8, immunosuppression and previous skin lesions (eg Bowen's disease and solar keratosis).

- When these lesions arise in a chronic venous ulcer this is termed a Marjolin's ulcer. These tend not to be as aggressive as spontaneous SCC, but should also be treated vigorously once they have been confirmed by biopsy.

- Treatment of the primary lesion is by wide excision (1 cm margin).

- Palpable nodes are treated by means of en bloc lymph-node dissection or, more recently, by sentinel-node mapping, to confirm histological involvement. Many patients with SCC have enlarged nodes, but these are due to reactive changes in up to one-third of cases.

- Radiotherapy is of unproven benefit, and chemotherapy has no role.

General

**CASE
39**

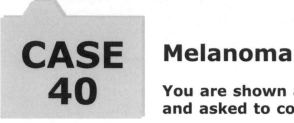

CASE 40

Melanoma

You are shown a pigmented lesion and asked to comment on it.

This melanoblastic tumour is the commonest cancer in young adults between the ages of 20 and 39 years, and it has a poor prognosis in those with nodal or distant-organ disease. It may develop in the skin, eye or brain, and its incidence is increasing.

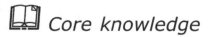 Core knowledge

The features of a pigmented lesion which suggest malignancy include the following:

- increase in size
- ulceration
- change in colour
- irritation
- bleeding
- halo of pigmentation
- satellite nodules
- enlarged local lymph nodes
- evidence of distant spread.

Exposure to sunlight is the most common initiating event with regard to the proliferation of melanoma. Men are most commonly affected on the back, chest and upper limbs, while women are most frequently affected on the back, upper extremities and lower extremities.

General

The classification of melanoma is important, as each subtype has a varying prognosis.

- Superficial spreading: this is the commonest type, accounting for 70% of cases. The tumour has irregular borders with a varied colour pattern and a generally good prognosis by stage of disease.
- Nodular: this accounts for about 15% of cases, with a peak incidence in the sixth decade of life. The tumour is generally dark blue or black. This type exhibits a vertical growth phase, with rapid dermal invasion, and the prognosis is generally poor.
- Acral, lentiginous and mucosal: these account for 10% of cases, and are generally black but can also be amelanotic. They grow slowly in a radial direction, and their prognosis is intermediate between those of the above two types.
- Lentigo maligna (Hutchinson's freckle): this is the least common type, and it occurs in older patients. The tumour grows radially and vertical extension is infrequent. It has an excellent prognosis.

Staging is done by one of three methods:

1 Clark's level of invasion (pathological)

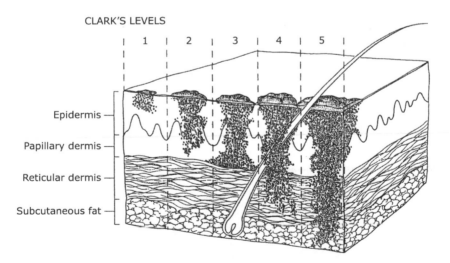

Fig 13 Clark's levels

General

CASE
40

2 Breslow's thickness (pathological)

3 AJCC staging (clinical)

You must be familiar with these staging procedures.

Discussion points

- The differential diagnoses include benign naevi, seborrhoeic keratoses, and simple freckles and pigmented basal-cell carcinomas.

- Predisposing factors include exposure to sunlight, a positive family history, xeroderma pigmentosum, dysplastic naevus syndrome (the risk of developing melanoma is 100% if two family members are affected), experiencing sunburn as a child, and pre-existing skin lesions or previous melanoma.

- The prognosis is related to depth of invasion.

Advanced knowledge

Margins for lesions depend on thickness:

< 1.5 mm	1 cm margin
1.5–4.0 mm	2 cm margin
> 4.0 mm	3 cm margin

Primary treatment consists of surgical excision. Treatment includes intralesional BCG therapy, which is good for satellitosis and cutaneous metastases, as well as immunotherapy, in the form of vaccines to promote the formation of anti-tumour antibodies, and interferon for nodal (Stage III) disease.

General

**CASE
40**

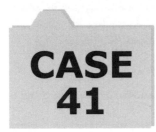

Skin grafts

You are brought to a patient with a skin graft on their leg at the site of a previous wide excision of a squamous-cell carcinoma.

The essential points to convey in this case are an understanding of tissue coverage and the use of grafts in reconstructive surgery.

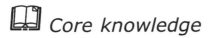

Core knowledge

Skin grafts are segments of epidermis and dermis that have been detached from their native blood supply to be transplanted to another area of the body where skin coverage is required. These may be autografts (from another part of the same person), allografts (from a different person but the same species, probably cadaveric) or xenografts (from a different species, usually a pig). Skin can now also be cultured in the laboratory from tissue-engineered human epidermal cells. This is especially useful for burn victims.

There are various types of graft, including the following.

- Split-thickness grafts contain the epidermis and a portion of dermis. The abdomen, buttocks and thighs are the commonest donor sites. These grafts are useful for covering large areas, are easy to harvest, and the donor site can be reused following re-epithelialisation within 10–14 days. However, they are not very durable, and they give an inferior cosmetic result to full-thickness grafts because they contract more after placement.

- Full-thickness grafts contain the epidermis and the full dermis without subcutaneous fat. They are most useful for covering defects in the face or hand, where a flap is unsuitable. The donor site should be matched as closely as possible for pigment- and hair-bearing characteristics. The disadvantages are that the donor site is prone to primary contracture and there is a limited number of donor sites.

- Composite grafts contain multiple tissues (eg a fingertip or an earlobe). They can be successful in young patients or in cases where a good blood supply is available.

General

Grafts will fail if they are placed on exposed bone, tendon or cartilage without their respective fascial coverings. Moreover, they will not 'take' on infected, necrotic or irradiated tissue.

Grafts are harvested either in the traditional manner with hand-held knives such as the Humby or Weck knife, or with powered dermatomes.

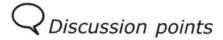

Discussion points

Care of the recipient and donor sites is necessary to prevent infection and movement at the transfer site.

General

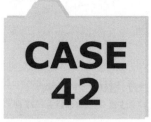

CASE 42

Flaps

A skin flap consists of tissues that have been transferred from one site to another while maintaining a continuous blood supply through a vascular pedicle.

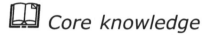 *Core knowledge*

Because of their intrinsic blood supply, flaps are useful for healing and for covering defects that require padding. They are indicated to cover areas with exposed cartilage, open joints, bare cortical bone or bare tendon, and if the viability of the recipient area has been depressed by scanning or radiotherapy.

Types include:

- Local flaps to repair skin defects by local V–Y or Z-plasty adjustments.
- Pedicle vascular flap (retaining its vascular or neurovascular oxide pedicle). An example includes the deltopectoral flap which is based on the perforating branches of the internal mammary artery.
- Myocuteneous flaps. These are used to cover large defects of tissue or for breast reconstruction. Examples include the latissimus dense flap or the transverse rectus abdominus muscle (TRAM) flap.

General

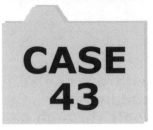

CASE 43

Hydradenitis suppurativa

Examine the axillae of this man. What do you think these lesions are?

Hydradenitis suppurativa is an infection of the apocrine sweat glands that most commonly affects the axillae, but can also affect the groin and perianal region. Women are more commonly affected than men. In the perianal region it can mimic fistula in ano. Wherever it occurs, the treatment of choice is wide local excision, but it often recurs.

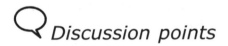

The examination

Most of the signs are visible on inspection alone. The axillary skin is usually heavily scarred and multiple sinuses are present. The major complication of these lesions is superficial infection leading to pain and pyrexia.

Tell the examiner that you would like to examine the groin area and enquire about systemic illnesses such as diabetes mellitus.

Discussion points

- The primary treatment is to eradicate infection with antibiotic therapy or drainage, if abscesses are present.
- Excision of the affected areas is not always successful, and skin grafting may be required to provide skin coverage of large defects.

After introducing yourself and washing your hands, inspect the patient from the front.

General

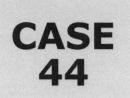

CASE 44

Neck swelling – general approach

Examine this man's neck.

🔍 *The examination*

Inspect for any visible lumps, noting their characteristics as described previously. Then ask the patient to open their mouth and stick their tongue out. If this is a thyroglossal cyst, it will move upward on tongue protrusion. This can be a difficult sign to elicit. Thyroid swellings do not move on protrusion of the tongue, but both types of swelling can move on swallowing.

Next ask the patient to swallow, using the glass of water that is provided. Direct the patient to take a sip, hold it in their mouth and swallow when asked to do so.

Palpation is best performed from behind and should be approached systematically. If a lump is palpable, relate its anatomical location to the examiner and gently use your fingertips to elicit the physical signs. Using the information you have elicited, answer the following questions.

- Is it mid-line or lateral?
- Is it solid or cystic?
- Are the features benign or malignant?

General

CASE
44

Discussion points

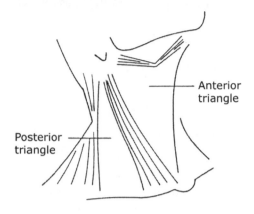

Fig 14 Anatomical triangles of the neck

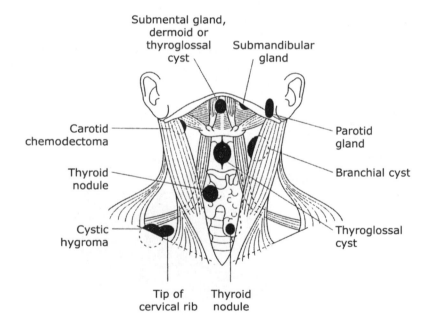

Fig 15 Lumps in the neck

CASE
44

There are many causes of neck swellings, which are discussed in detail in the following cases. They can be summarised as follows.

- Midline

    Thyroid swelling

    Thyroglossal cyst
- Lateral anterior triangle

    Lymph nodes

    Chemodectoma

    Branchial cyst

    Cold abscess (TB)
- Lateral posterior triangle

    Lymph nodes

    Pharyngeal pouch

    Cystic hygroma
- Sternocleidomastoid (SCM)

    SCM tumour.

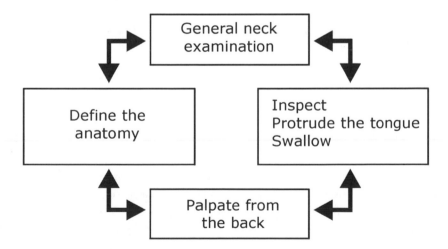

Fig 16 Approach to neck examination

CASE
44

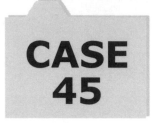

CASE 45

Thyroglossal cyst

Examine this man's neck.

As outlined previously, you will need a systematic approach to lumps in the neck or elsewhere. Thyroglossal cysts are remnants of the thyroglossal duct, which begins at the foramen caecum of the tongue. When the duct or a portion of it fails to obliterate, a cyst is formed.

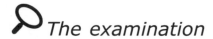

The examination

Examine the patient as described previously. Inspection will reveal a small cyst in the mid-line of the neck. Most are seen either just above the hyoid bone or between the hyoid bone and the isthmus of the thyroid gland.

The overlying skin will appear normal unless there is infection. Infection in the cyst may also cause a sinus to develop, leading to pain, tenderness to palpation and an increase in size. The cysts appear smooth and spherical. Because of their obvious location, these cysts can cause cosmetic problems while they are still very small.

Palpation will usually reveal a fluctuant cyst that moves from side to side. Protrusion of the tongue causes elevation of a thyroglossal cyst.

Most thyroglossal cysts present in adult life, usually in the fourth decade. They rarely present at birth, and they tend to cause problems with cosmesis rather than any other symptoms.

Sistrunk's operation involves removing the sinus tract (if present) and the cyst. Most surgeons excise the central portion of the hyoid bone and then follow the tract up to the level of the foramen caecum. The incidence of recurrence is higher if the hyoid is not excised.

Histologically, thyroglossal cysts may contain ectopic thyroid tissue that can undergo malignant change to papillary carcinoma.

General

CASE
45

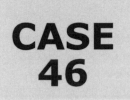

CASE 46

Cervical lymphadenopathy

Examine this man's neck.

This is a common scenario both in examinations and in clinical practice. Cervical lymphadenopathy is the commonest reason for a neck swelling, and there are four main causes:

- Lymphoma
- primary or secondary (head and neck, thorax, abdomen, breast) tumours
- infection
- leukaemias
- sarcoidosis.

⌕ The examination

The neck examination is easily assessed in exams. Approach this case in the same manner as before. Inspect the patient, and ask them to swallow and then to stick their tongue out. Next palpate the glands systematically after informing the patient that this is what you intend to do. By convention, this is done from behind the patient, beginning with the submental group, and progressing to the submandibular, the jugulodigastric, parotid and pre-auricular, down the neck to the anterior cervical chain, then the supraclavicular, back up the posterior neck to the postauricular and finally to the occipital group of nodes.

This procedure can be facilitated by flexing the neck slightly to allow relaxation of the anterior neck musculature. You can also move to the front and examine the suspected lymph node from that position.

The features of enlarged lymph nodes are that they are commonly multiple, they have a firm or shotty consistency in infection or leukaemic disorders, and they may be either fixed to skin or matted together in metastatic disease.

If you think that these are reactive nodes due to infection, state that you would perform a full head and neck examination to look for a focus. If you think that they are suggestive of malignancy, offer to examine the breast and the thyroid gland. The liver and spleen may be enlarged in lymphoma or leukaemia.

General

Q Discussion points

The investigation of cervical lymphadenopathy includes haematological indices to check for erythrocyte sedimentation rate, full blood count and C-reactive protein (non-specific indicators of an acute-phase response). Biochemical investigations should include thyroid function tests and angiotensin-converting enzyme (ACE) levels, which are often raised in infiltrative diseases such as sarcoidosis.

Imaging modalities such as ultrasound (solid or cystic), CT or MRI (which demonstrates metastatic involvement and may detect other subclinical lymphadenopathy or primary lesions) are all useful.

Fine-needle aspiration cytology is useful but does not allow tissue architecture to be studied, and is limited by the skill of the cytologist who interprets it. An open biopsy will allow tissue architecture to be evaluated.

Metastatic lymph nodes

- These are the commonest cause of lymphadenopathy in adults.
- The primary is often located in the oral cavity or larynx.
- Most patients are over 55 years of age, although papillary thyroid carcinoma may be present in patients in their twenties.
- Other systemic symptoms include weight loss, hoarseness, dyspnoea, etc.
- An enlarged left supraclavicular node is called Virchow's node. When present, it is Troisier's sign.
- Metastatic tumour deposits make the nodes feel hard.

Primary lymph node malignancies

- Most are lymphomas (Hodgkin's or non-Hodgkin's).
- They are often associated with systemic symptoms such as malaise, weight loss and fever (Pel–Ebstein fever).
- Nodes are smooth to the touch and rubbery in consistency.
- They have a much younger age of onset than secondary nodal cancers.

General

CASE 46

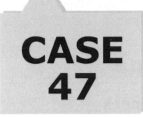

CASE 47

Cystic hygroma

Examine this man's neck.

These cases are difficult to find for adult surgical examinations, and are more likely to be encountered in a paediatric examination. Cystic hygromata are collections of lymphatic sacs filled with clear lymph fluid. They commonly occur at the root of the neck, or at the junction between the arms and the head and neck.

The examination

The general neck examination has already been described. Points that are specific to cystic hygromata include the following:

- They are usually found at the base of the posterior triangle.
- They transilluminate brilliantly.
- They are soft, fluctuant and compressible.
- They usually present in childhood, but may present later.

Some cystic hygromata can be very large and extend throughout the whole of the base of the neck. It is vital to perform a thorough examination of the oropharynx, as large cysts can extend into the retropharyngeal space.

Discussion points

- Complications of cystic hygromata include respiratory or gastrointestinal obstruction in the perinatal period, and cosmetic problems in childhood or early adulthood.
- Treatment consists of surgical excision.

General

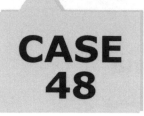

CASE 48

Chemodectoma

Examine this man's neck.

General

Chemodectomas are rare tumours of the chemoreceptor tissue in the carotid body. They are usually benign, but may occasionally become quite large and undergo malignant change. The lump is painless, sometimes pulsatile, and extremely slow growing, so much so that the patient may be unaware of it. The age of onset is between 40 and 60 years. Chemodectomas may be bilateral.

The examination

Palpation in this area can induce a vasovagal attack due to pressure on the carotid bifurcation, so be gentle! The carotid bifurcation is at or just below the level of the hyoid bone, so chemodectomas are found above this, beneath the anterior edge of the stenocleidomastoid muscle.

These tumours are closely related to the carotid arteries and therefore only move from side to side, not up and down.

They may be pulsatile due to any of the following:

- a very vascular tumour
- the external carotid artery running across the tumour
- a transmitted pulsation from the internal carotid artery.

Remember to check the other side, as the tumour could be bilateral.

Enquire about syncopal attacks, transient ischaemic attacks and neurological symptoms.

The major differential diagnosis is cervical lymphadenopathy, so it is important to exclude generalised lymphadenopathy.

Q Discussion points

- Investigations include duplex ultrasonography or angiography (which shows the classic appearance of splaying of the carotid bifurcation).

- Surgical excision with pre-operative embolisation is widely practised, and in certain cases local fractionated radiotherapy is helpful.

General

CASE
48

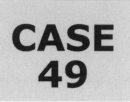

CASE 49

Branchial cyst

Examine this man's neck.

Branchial cysts are remnants of the branchial clefts, usually the second one. They are developmental abnormalities, but often do not present until late in adult life. They are lined by squamous epithelium and can be prone to infection and sinus formation. They occur higher in the neck than carotid body tumours.

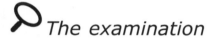 *The examination*

The general neck examination has already been described. The specific features of branchial cysts are as follows.

- Most present at between 15 and 25 years of age.
- There is no gender predominance.
- They occur in the anterior triangle of neck opposite the upper or middle third of the sternocleidomastoid (SCM).
- They are usually painless unless infected.
- They are fluctuant, but difficult to demonstrate if small.
- A fistulous opening may be visible.
- They are usually opaque when transilluminated.

☁ *Discussion points*

A cyst is an abnormal collection in a sac lined by epithelium.

A sinus is a blind-ending tract that opens out onto an epithelial surface and is lined by epithelium or granulation tissue.

A fistula is an abnormal connection between two epithelial surfaces.

- Be concise in these definitions. A branchial sinus may be seen as a small dimple in the skin at the junction of the middle and lower third of the SCM. The skin opening is accentuated by swallowing.
- Treatment consists of surgical excision. Recurrence rates are higher in the presence of infection.
- Sometimes the fluid in the cyst contains cholesterol crystals secreted by the sebaceous glands in the epithelial lining.

As this is a frequent cause of surgical admission, these cases are commonly encountered in examinations.

General

CASE 49

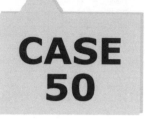

CASE 50

Cellulitis

Examine this woman's leg.

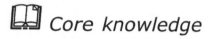 Core knowledge

Cellulitis is inflammation of the dermal and subcutaneous tissues secondary to non-suppurative bacterial invasion. It often results from a puncture wound or a similar breach in the skin. In the lower limb, the main differential diagnoses are deep vein thrombosis or secondary infection of dependent oedema or lymphoedema.

Cellulitis is characterised by redness, oedema and localised tenderness.

The examination

On inspection, there will be redness and oedema of the affected area. It will be tender to the touch and the oedema may be pitting. On admission, house officers will often delineate the extent of the cellulitis, and this can be used to determine whether the condition is improving or not. When the cellulitis is resolving, the skin becomes less tense and wrinkles appear. Blisters, if present, usually release a serous discharge.

If the regional lymphatics are involved, there may be red tender streaks leading to the draining lymph nodes.

$\mathcal{Q}$ *Discussion points*

- The commonest causative organisms are streptococci, which will usually respond to a combination of benzylpenicillin and flucloxacillin. If the patient does not respond, you should consider the possibility that there may be an underlying deep-seated abscess.

- There may also be a pyrexia, and a full blood count often shows a neutrophilic leukocytosis.

Urology

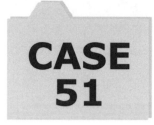

CASE 51

Scrotal examination – general approach

Examine this man's scrotum.

There are a number of scrotal abnormalities which are available to examiners as OSCE or short cases, including hydrocoele, varicocoele, epididymal cysts, and testicular swellings such as testicular carcinoma. These should not be confused with groin swellings such as hernias, which are their main differential diagnosis. The patient should be examined both lying and standing, and exposure is critical.

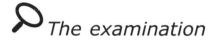

The examination

Look

- Does the swelling arise from the scrotum or the groin? Can you get above it?

- Look for surgical incisions. These can be difficult to see, and may be hidden in the groin creases or in the median raphe between the two hemiscrotums.

Feel

- Palpate the testes one at a time, deciding on the contour and consistency, and looking for any lumps or irregularities.

- Is the lump separate from the testis and epididymis?

- Does it transilluminate?

- Examine the inguinal nodes (which are enlarged in processes involving the scrotal skin or the penis) and the rest of the abdomen and groin. A useful algorithm is shown in Fig 17.

Urology

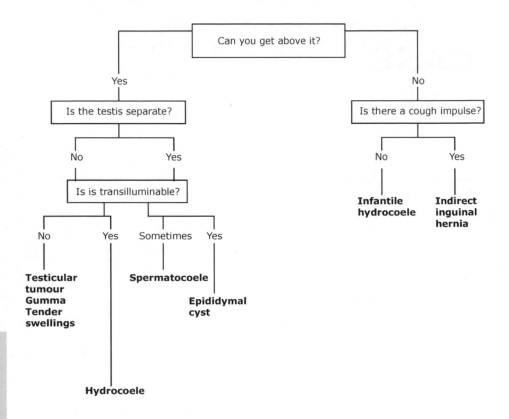

Fig 17 Algorithm for scrotal examination

Urology

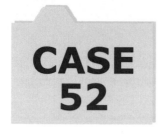

Hydrocoele

Examine this man's scrotum.

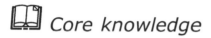 *Core knowledge*

A hydrocoele is a fluctuant and transilluminable swelling that cannot be felt separately from the testis. Hydrocoeles can be extremely large and result from a patent processus vaginalis. There are four types.

- **Vaginal hydrocoeles** are the commonest type. They occur because the fluid accumulates in the tunica vaginalis surrounding the testis but does not extend up the cord. They do not communicate with the peritoneal cavity, and are often associated with infection or testicular tumours. This is important, as up to 10% of testicular malignancies present with a hydrocoele.

- **Hydrocoeles of the cord** occur because fluid accumulates around the spermatic cord, and the mass may appear anywhere along the cord, often around the ductus deferens. They can be difficult to distinguish from an irreducible inguinal hernia, but are separate from the testis. When in doubt, gentle traction on the testis will pull a hydrocoele of the cord down and make the diagnosis clear.

- **Congenital hydrocoeles** occur because the proximal portion of the processus vaginalis has failed to obliterate, and the hydrocoele is filled with peritoneal fluid as the sac communicates with the peritoneal cavity. This type is commonly found in children under the age of 3 years.

- **Infantile hydrocoeles** occur due to incomplete resorption of the fluid from the tunica vaginalis after the processus has sealed off. They do not communicate with the peritoneal cavity and can present at any age.

The examination

Apply the knowledge gained in the previous question and perform the examination as directed.

Urology

Q *Discussion points*

The treatment of hydrocoeles depends on the symptomatology associated with them. Even if they are asymptomatic, the presence of an associated malignancy should be excluded by clinical examination and testicular ultrasound. The choices range from careful observation to aspiration of peritoneal fluid if the hydrocoele is large or interfering with urinary or sexual function, or ultimately surgical intervention.

The operative treatment is either a Lord's procedure, in which the sac is plicated with interrupted sutures to the junction of the epididymis and the testis, or Jaboulay's operation, in which the excess sac is excised and the remainder is replaced behind the cord. These procedures are both achieved via scrotal incisions.

Vaginal hydrocoeles are commonly associated with testicular malignancy, orchitis, torsion following inguinal hernia repair, or any type of scrotal trauma.

Urology

CASE 52

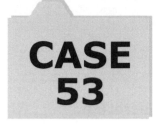

CASE 53

Epididymal cyst

Examine this man's scrotum.

You should proceed as described for the previous cases.

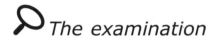

The examination

Epididymal cysts are usually small, and in most cases there will be no visual scrotal abnormality. They are brilliantly transilluminable and are separate from the testis. However, if they contain sperm, they are not transilluminable and are termed spermatocoeles. They are separate from the testis and distinct from the superficial inguinal ring (ie you can get above the swelling). Complete your examination by inspecting the contralateral hemiscrotum.

Discussion points

- Management of these cysts consists of leaving them alone unless they are large or painful. If they are symptomatic, they can be excised. Surgery carries an appreciable risk of post-operative fibrosis, leading to subfertility.

- With the increase in vasectomy rates, there is now a higher incidence of spermatocoeles. These can be treated in a similar manner.

Urology

CASE 53

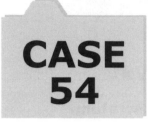

CASE 54

Varicocoele

Examine this man's scrotum.

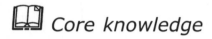 Core knowledge

This scrotal abnormality is said to resemble 'a bag of worms', and is caused by an abnormal dilatation and elongation of the pampiniform venous plexus. Varicocoeles can only be felt with the patient standing up, and on inspection there may be no visible abnormality apart from the fact that the contralateral testis may appear to sit higher.

They occur predominantly on the left side. This is probably due to a combination of factors. The pampiniform plexus drains into the testicular vein, which is longer on the left side and frequently lacks a terminal valve to prevent backflow in the vein, and the left renal vein may be compressed by the colon.

The examination

On inspection there may be no scrotal abnormality. On palpation there will be no abnormality unless the patient is examined while standing.

Varicocoeles have the following characteristics.

- They do not transilluminate.
- They are separate from the testis.
- They are distinct from the superficial inguinal ring.
- There may be a cough impulse.

As always, remember to examine the other hemiscrotum.

Urology

Q *Discussion points*

- In older men, beware the varicocoele that does not disappear on lying down. This may signify the presence of retroperitoneal disease, especially renal-cell carcinoma, causing occlusion of the left renal vein.

- There are several postulated reasons why almost all varicocoeles occur on the left side, as has already been discussed.

- Varicocoeles get worse with age, and there is a small risk of subfertility problems.

- Surgery can be performed either by a minimally invasive approach, using laparoscopic ligation of the veins in the inguinal canal, or by an open approach in the same area. The Palomo operation, which consists of high ligation of the testicular vein in the retroperitoneum, is also employed.

Urology

CASE 54

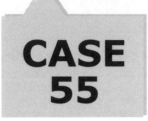

CASE 55

Testicular tumour

Examine this man's scrotum.

Testicular tumours are the commonest solid tumours in the 15 to 35 years age group, with a lifetime risk of 1 in 500. The associated mortality is now around 10% with effective multimodality therapy. Testicular ultrasound examination is mandatory, and is sensitive for the identification of a hypoechoic lesion. Serum tumour markers, $\alpha-$ fetoprotein and β-human chorionic gonadotrophin, can aid diagnosis of the tumour type, and are also useful for monitoring the response to treatment.

The examination

The typical clinical finding is of a painless testicular mass. On inspection, a testicular swelling may be visible, especially if there is an associated hydrocoele. On palpation, there are several diagnostic features.

- The swelling is inseparable from the testis.
- It is hard and irregular.
- It will not transilluminate.
- It is non-tender.
- It is distinct from the superficial inguinal ring.
- It may have an associated hydrocoele.

Demonstrate these features and examine the patient for lymphadenopathy in the abdominal region. There will be no inguinal lymphadenopathy unless the scrotum is involved. The para-aortic nodes are most commonly involved, and these are impalpable unless they are grossly enlarged.

Testicular tumours commonly metastasise, and a thorough examination of the chest and abdomen, looking for pulmonary metastases and hepatic involvement, should be undertaken. Advise the examiner of your plan.

Urology

$\mathcal{Q}$ Discussion points

- The majority of testicular tumours are seminomatous (60%), and most of the non-seminomatous tumours are teratomas. The initial treatment is the same, namely radical inguinal orchidectomy with further therapy determined by tumour type and stage of disease. Seminomas are more radiosensitive than teratomas and have an older age of onset (usually the 30–40 years age group, compared with the 20–30 years age group for teratomas). Interestingly, tumour markers are usually normal in patients with seminomas, but are usually raised in those with teratomas.

- The presentation is normally that of a painless mass or a dull ache in one testicle in a young man. It is often discovered following an incidental episode of testicular trauma. Acute pain is uncommon but may mimic testicular torsion, and back pain may reflect para-aortic nodal involvement.

- Other benign conditions can mimic testicular tumours, such as orchitis, chronic infection or calcification in an established hydrocoele.

- Surgery is performed by an inguinal approach with lymphovascular ligation prior to mobilisation of the testis, to prevent dispersal of viable tumour cells into the circulation.

Urology

CASE 55

CASE 56

Transplanted kidney

Examine the abdomen of this patient.

This scenario is commonly encountered in exam short cases and OSCEs. The key is for candidates to understand the pathophysiology of renal failure, the stigmata of chronic renal insufficiency and the basic principles of renal transplantation.

The examination

Most patients with functioning renal transplants will be on immunosuppression, and almost all of them will have had a lengthy period of peritoneal dialysis or haemodialysis. There may be evidence of steroid therapy with cutaneous ecchymoses or paper-thin skin. The radial or brachial arteries may have been used as sites for fashioning of arteriovenous fistulae (see Vascular disorders section) by the Brescia–Cimino procedure.

In the abdomen itself there will be a distinctive scar in the right or left iliac fossa termed a Rutherford–Morrison incision, which allows extraperitoneal placement of the transplanted kidney. Look for the presence of scars on the abdomen from previous tunneled CAPD (continuous ambulatory peritoneal dialysis) catheter placement (Tenckhoff catheter) or a loin incision from a nephrectomy.

Beneath the iliac incision there will be a well-circumscribed and superficial mass. Remember that the transplanted kidney is extraperitoneal and the two non-functioning kidneys are retroperitoneal. The ureter is anastomosed to the bladder and the arterial supply and venous drainage to the external iliac vessels.

Urology

$\bigcirc$ Discussion points

- Renal transplant is now performed routinely. The most common indications are end-stage renal disease due to diabetic nephropathy, polycystic kidneys, hypertensive nephropathy or glomerulonephritis.

- Transplant immunology is complex, but matching of donor to recipient is based on ABO compatibility and human leukocyte antigen (HLA) compatibility. The HLA DR locus is the most important one, followed by the B and A loci. The graft survival rate at 1 year is 90% in patients who are appropriately ABO and HLA matched.

- Transplant rejection is a serious complication. It is avoided by the use of immunosuppressive drugs such as steroids or cyclosporin.

- Hyperacute rejection occurs within hours of surgery and is due to pre-formed antibodies in a sensitised recipient. The activation of memory T-cells is a secondary immune response that occurs between 1 and 4 days post-operatively, leading to accelerated acute rejection. In acute rejection, a cell-mediated response occurs in which renal epithelial cells are destroyed by a lymphocytic interstitial infiltrate. This typically happens between 5 days and 2 weeks after surgery. Chronic rejection differs from acute rejection in that humoral immunity mediates the response. It occurs around 2 weeks after surgery.

- The clinical features of graft rejection are a reduction in urine output, marked graft tenderness and a rising creatinine concentration.

Urology

CASE
56

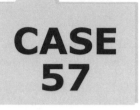

CASE 57

Enlarged kidney

Examine the abdomen of this patient.

Urology

Examination of the kidneys is difficult, and renal enlargement is difficult to demonstrate or quantify clinically using ballottement. Nevertheless, it is an important clinical skill and one that is often tested as part of the overall abdominal examination. The causes of renal enlargement are myriad.

☌ The examination

Inspection rarely reveals anything of note, but there may be associated supraclavicular lymphadenopathy if the cause of the enlargement is an advanced renal tumour. In normal individuals the lower pole of the right kidney is often palpable. On the left, the kidney must be differentiated from the spleen, and on the right, from an enlarged liver or distended gallbladder. The following features aid this distinction.

- Kidneys are ballottable (bimanually palpable).
- Kidneys descend vertically with respiration.
- The examining hand can, in theory, get above the swelling when the latter is of renal origin.

Ballottement of the kidneys is a difficult clinical skill to acquire, and is often inexpertly practised. The anatomy of the renal triangle is straightforward, and the ballotting hand (posterior) should aim to tip the kidney anteriorly to be felt by the anterior hand at the peak of inspiration. It is difficult to trap the kidney between the two hands, and only basic information on size and texture is usually discernible.

Q Discussion points

There are many causes of renal enlargement, of which the following are most common.

Congenital causes

- Polycystic kidney disease
- Horseshoe kidney
- Hypertrophied single kidney.

Acquired causes

- Renal neoplasms
- Renal cysts
- Hydronephrosis
- Pyonephrosis/perinephric abscess
- Renal vein thrombosis.

Renal cysts are very common, and are present in around 50% of all people over 50 years of age. The majority are asymptomatic.

Renal-cell carcinomas are relatively common, and most are less than 3 cm in diameter. Historically, they presented with the triad of loin pain, haematuria and a flank mass. Nowadays, most are incidental discoveries on abdominal imaging performed for another reason. They are frequently associated with paraneoplastic syndromes. They may also present with left-sided varicocoele.

Urology

CASE
57

Endocrine disorders

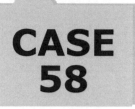

CASE 58

Thyroid examination – general approach

Examine this man's neck.

Patients with mid-line neck swellings will commonly have thyroid pathology. The same rules apply as in Case 44. You are directed to examine the neck and will probably not have the opportunity to ask specific questions. Introduce yourself (note whether the patient is hoarse – recurrent laryngeal nerve [RLN] palsy) and shake hands (note whether they are diaphoretic – hyperthyroid).

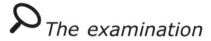

The examination

Inspect

- A goitre may be obvious if present.
- Is the swelling localised to one side or global?
- Does the patient look hypothyroid, euthyroid or hyperthyroid?

Swallow

- There will be a glass of water, often out of view.
- On swallowing, does the swelling move? If it does, it is a thyroid swelling.
- Ask the patient to stick their tongue out. A thyroglossal cyst will move upward.
- Note the shape of the gland on movement.
- Can the inferior border be seen? If not, it may be retrosternal.
- Are there scars around the neck from previous surgery?
- Are there dilated veins from possible thoracic inlet obstruction, if the gland extends retrosternally?

Endocrine disorders

CASE 58

Palpate

- Move **behind** the patient, reposition them if necessary and slightly flex the neck to relax the sternocleidomastoid. Use the finger pulps to palpate the H-shaped gland.
- Can you estimate the size?
- Can you feel the lower border?
- Ask the patient to swallow again.
- Is there just one nodule or is the whole gland nodular?
- Is the gland tender, soft, firm or hard?
- Is it mobile or tethered to skin?
- Is there a palpable thrill? This is a sign of thyrotoxicosis.
- Is there cervical lymphadenopathy (thyroid neoplasm)?
- Is the carotid pulsation normal? It can be diminished in neoplastic infiltration.
- Move to the front and palpate the gland again with the thumbs. Is there tracheal displacement?

Percuss

Percuss from the manubriosternal joint upward and from side to side. A dull note may signify a retrosternal goitre.

Auscultate

A bruit can be due to hyperthyroidism causing a metabolically overactive gland. Rule out a venous hum with pressure over the neck base and a carotid bruit, which is louder in the lateral neck, over the carotid itself.

Pemberton's sign

This is a test for thoracic inlet obstruction caused by a retrosternal goitre or any other mediastinal mass. Ask the patient to raise their arms above their head from the side. The venous congestion which this induces when positive leads to plethora and cyanosis, which may be associated with inspiratory stridor. It is important to be aware that this can also induce syncope.

The commonest causes of diffuse thyroid enlargement are Grave's disease if the patient is hyperthyroid, and simple colloid goitre or thyroiditis if they are euthyroid. Thyroiditis can also cause the gland to be tender.

The commonest cause of nodular enlargement is a true solitary thyroid nodule (see Case 59) or a multinodular goitre (see Case 60).

**CASE
58**

Endocrine disorders

Q Discussion points

- Make sure that you are au fait with the eye and hand signs of thyroid disease.

Eye signs

- Hair loss from outer third of the eyebrow (hypothyroidism)
- Thyrotoxicosis
  - Lid lag
  - Lid retraction
  - Proptosis
  - Exophthalmos
  - Chemosis
  - Opthalmoplegia

Hand signs

- Diaphoresis
- Palmar erythema
- Thyroid acropachy
- Arrhythmia
- Fine tremor
- Ophthalmoplegia
- Vitiligo
- Plummer's nails
  - onycholysis

Endocrine disorders

CASE
58

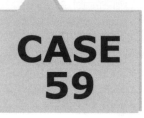

CASE 59

Solitary thyroid nodule

Examine this man's neck.

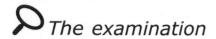

The examination

The examination is as outlined previously in Case 58. About 50% of all true solitary thyroid nodules are malignant in the young and the elderly. The causes of a solitary thyroid nodule are summarised below.

Benign causes

- Dominant nodule in a multinodular goitre
- Bleeding into a colloid cyst or nodule
- Simple cyst (very rare)
- Follicular adenoma.

Malignant causes

- Thyroid carcinoma
- Metastases
- Lymphoma (rare).

Thyroid nodules are palpable, move on swallowing but not on tongue protrusion, and are often malignant, so check for lymphadenopathy. Although the nodule may feel solitary, in fact up to 50% of all patients with a solitary nodule have a multinodular goitre.

Endocrine disorders

Q *Discussion points*

- Solitary nodules are more common in women, and usually occur in the fourth and fifth decades of life. About 10% of those that occur in middle age are malignant, but this figure rises to 50% in the young and the elderly. Thyrotoxicosis caused by a solitary thyroid nodule is rare, and is almost never malignant.

- Clinical examination is unreliable for determining the cause, and examination must be accompanied by cytological assessment, a technetium scan and neck ultrasound.

Endocrine disorders

**CASE
59**

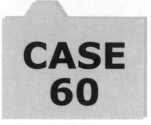

Multinodular goitre

Examine this man's neck.

🔍 *The examination*

The approach and examination are as described previously (Case 58). The gland should be easily palpable, but perform the thyroid examination as before. There may be a dominant nodule within the substance of the gland. Also check for tracheal displacement and evidence of retrosternal extension.

Atrial fibrillation is seen in up to 50% of all patients with multinodular goitre (MNG). MNG can be caused by goitrogens, dyshormonogenesis, iodine deficiency or autoimmune causes.

Clinical features of MNG

- Positive family history
- No eye signs
- Same aetiology as simple colloid goitre
- Mainly affects middle-aged women
- Can sometimes lead to mild hyperthyroidism.

Multinodular goitres are common, and most of them do not require any treatment. If the patient has compression symptoms or new-onset hyperthyroidism, or is concerned about cosmetic issues, MNG can be investigated with thyroid function tests to rule out hyperthroidism, ultrasound examination to determine the extent of the cysts, and a technetium scan to determine whether or not the nodules are functioning (ie hot or cold).

Investigation is needed if there is any suspicion of malignancy or a dominant nodule in the gland.

Treatment is a surgical subtotal thyroidectomy which has the advantage that it does not put the parathyroid glands at risk. It is offered to patients with compression-type symptoms, retrosternal extension or problems with cosmetic issues.

Endocrine disorders

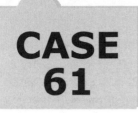

Simple colloid goitre

Examine this man's neck.

Examine the gland and neck in the same order as before (Case 58), and note the difference in the clinical examination. This condition is due to low levels of circulating thyroid hormone leading to an excess of thyroid-stimulating hormone (TSH), which causes the gland to enlarge. The commonest pathological cause is iodine deficiency, but physiological causes include pregnancy and puberty. The term 'colloid goitre' is used to describe the late stage of diffuse hyperplasia. The acini are distended with colloid that has not been released because the TSH levels have decreased and the gland is no longer stimulated. The patient will usually be euthyroid.

Simple colloid goitre and thyroiditis (Hashimoto's disease, Riedel's thyroiditis and De Quervain's thyroiditis, etc) all cause diffuse thyroid enlargement, as does Graves' disease. In diffuse enlargement due to thyroiditis the gland is often tender, and in Graves' disease it will be thyrotoxic.

🔍 *The examination*

The gland is diffusely enlarged with an absence of palpable nodules and may be extremely large. It is not usually tender on palpation. If the cause is physiological, the gland will not reach the same size as when the cause is iodine deficiency. The surface is usually smooth, but may become nodular over a period of many years. As before, check for tracheal deviation and retrosternal extension. There should be no eye signs, and the rest of the neck examination should be normal.

Endocrine disorders

CASE 61

Q *Discussion points*

- The simple colloid goitre is the commonest form of thyroid abnormality. It may occur in children in areas where goitre is endemic (so-called 'goitre belts'). In these areas, there is a deficiency of iodine in the drinking water. This iodine deficiency results in inadequate production of thyroid hormones, leading to hyperplasia due to overstimulation by TSH.

- Simple colloid goitres are more common in women than in men.

- Certain dietary factors cause dyshormogenesis. These are termed goitrogens, and they include cabbage and kale. The goitre appears slowly and is not usually associated with significant over- or under-activity of the gland. When the condition is longstanding, nodular changes develop in association with a change in the thyroid status.

- Treatment of symptomatic colloid goitres is by surgery, which is not without complications.

Complications of thyroidectomy

- Damage to recurrent laryngeal nerve – hoarseness
- Damage to parathyroid glands – hypocalcaemia
- Hypothyroidism
- Haemorrhage – if stridor develops, the wound must be opened
- Hyperthyroidism – thyroid storm
- Infection – uncommon.

Endocrine disorders

**CASE
61**

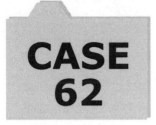

CASE 62

Thyroid history

This woman has a neck swelling. Ask her about her thyroid gland.

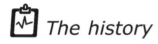 *The history*

The history of this patient's thyroid swelling should be used to assess the level of symptoms and the degree of lifestyle impairment, as well as to determine the status of the gland.

Ask about symptoms

- Is there a large, noticeable swelling? Is it unsightly to the patient?
- Are there problems with her voice/swallowing/breathing?
- Is the gland tender? This symptom is seen in thyroiditis or neoplasms.
- Is the patient hoarse? Neoplasms may infiltrate the recurrent laryngeal nerve (RLN), leading to cord paralysis.

Ask about the thyroid status

Symptoms of hyperthyroidism

- Hyperphagia with weight loss
- Dislikes warm weather
- Hot and sweaty
- Agitated, emotionally labile
- Fine tremor
- Arrhythmias – atrial fibrillation, tachycardia
- Proximal myopathy
- Prone to diarrhoea.

Endocrine disorders

CASE 62

Symptoms of hypothyroidism

- Weight gain, lethargy
- Dislikes cold weather
- Peaches-and-cream, dry skin
- Slowness of thought, depression
- Carpal tunnel syndrome
- Bradycardia
- Muscle fatigue
- Prone to constipation.

Also ask about the presence now and past history of eye symptoms, as well as previous surgery or medications. Use this information to decide whether the patient is euthyroid, hypothyroid or hyperthyroid.

CASE
62

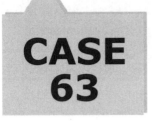

CASE 63

Salivary gland examination

Examine this man's neck.

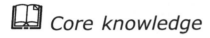

Core knowledge

The incidence of salivary gland swellings is decreasing, and they are no longer readily available for examinations, but are included here for the sake of completeness. The diseases that affect the salivary glands are uncommon. The surgical phenomena that we shall focus on are infections and calculi of the submandibular gland and tumours of the parotid gland. The medical conditions that affect the salivary glands are mumps and parotitis.

The function of the salivary glands is to produce saliva in response to food or neural stimuli.

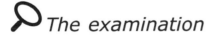

The examination

General points

Examine as for any lump and complete a full neck examination.

Specific points

The **submandibular gland** is located inferior to the mandibular ramus on the mylohyoid muscle, and its duct opens into the floor of the mouth. Submandibular calculi are relatively common due to the large amount of secretions and the close proximity to the oral cavity.

Submandibular calculi occur rarely in children, and there is no gender difference among young adults. The main symptoms are pain and swelling beneath the jaw, caused by obstruction of Wharton's duct. These symptoms appear or worsen during eating, and on examination you may be able to feel a swelling in the floor of the mouth with a gloved hand. With bimanual palpation you should be able to tell that the gland is outside the structures of the floor of the mouth.

Endocrine disorders

Unless the gland is infected, the overlying skin will be normal. The consistency of the gland will be rubbery hard when it is distended, and it does not transilluminate or reduce. The major differential diagnosis of submandibular gland swelling is deep cervical lymphadenopathy, and you should also examine the cervical lymph nodes.

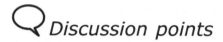 *Discussion points*

Generalised salivary gland enlargement can occur in autoimmune conditions such as Sjögren's syndrome.

Main features of Sjögren's syndrome

- Autoimmune aetiology
- More common in women than in men
- Includes any two of the following: xerostomia, keratoconjunctivitis sicca, connective tissue disease
- Is probably due to B-cell over-activation.

The **parotid gland** is more commonly affected by tumours than the submandibular gland, but can also be affected by infection and calculi. The commonest infection of the parotid gland is mumps, an epidemic viral parotitis that occurs mainly in children, giving bilateral painful swollen glands and the appearance of a 'double chin'. Mumps is the commonest cause of parotitis. The gland is located at the angle of the mandible and extends below and behind this landmark. Parotid swellings can easily be mistaken for enlarged upper deep cervical lymph nodes.

Endocrine disorders

CASE
63

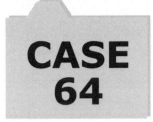

CASE 64

Gynaecomastia

Examine this man's chest.

Gynaecomastia is the commonest condition affecting the male breast, and is an enlargement of ductal and stromal tissues that are structurally different from the surrounding subcutaneous fat. The condition is entirely benign and usually reversible. Many cases will be idiopathic in apparently healthy men, but specific causes include hypogonadism, drugs, excess oestrogen and systemic diseases such as liver disease and thyrotoxicosis.

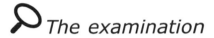

The examination

Presentation is usually with tender enlargement of the breast that is often unilateral. The patient may be concerned about the cosmetic appearance, pain or the possibility of an underlying malignancy.

Inspect the patient for the presence of unilateral or bilateral breast swellings.

Tell the examiner that you would like to examine the external genitalia and the nodal basins and look for clinical evidence of hepatic dysfunction or thyroid disease. Also enquire about the use of drugs (prescription or recreational).

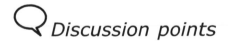

Discussion points

The causes of gynaecomastia are listed below.

- Increased oestrogens
    - Testicular tumours
    - Lung carcinoma
    - Liver disease
    - Adrenal disease
    - Thyrotoxicosis

Endocrine disorders

- Drug-induced causes

    Cannabis

    Cimetidine

    Digitalis

    Spironolactone

- Decreased androgens

    Renal failure

    Klinefelter's syndrome

    Viral orchitis

    Testicular feminisation.

Treatment consists of correction of the hormonal imbalance if present, or discontinuation of the causative drug if appropriate. Subcutaneous mastectomy is effective in cases where medical therapy fails or if there are psychological or cosmetic concerns.

Endocrine disorders

CASE
64

Vascular disorders

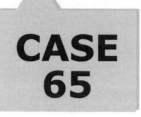

CASE 65

Diabetic foot

Examine the feet of this patient with diabetes.

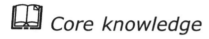 *Core knowledge*

Diabetes is a systemic disease, and it is rare to have unilateral limb findings in isolation. Because it begins in the small to medium-sized vessels, there will often have been multiple previous operations to remove metatarsal heads or digits if these have been affected by gangrene.

As there may also be a glove-and-stocking type neuropathy (especially in type 1 diabetes mellitus), there may be evidence of trauma or neuropathic ulcers secondary to insensate areas. Diabetes is one of the commonest causes of Charcot's joint, a progressive destructive joint neuropathy secondary to disturbed sensory innervation. This results in a painless deformed joint.

On clinical examination, the peripheral pulses are often present until late in the disease process and they commonly feel very prominent, probably due to vessel-wall hardening. Remember to ask the patient before palpating their feet, as they may well be painful.

Perform a neurological examination of the feet, working proximally to establish the level at which sensation returns to normal.

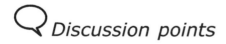 *Discussion points*

The examiner may ask you to continue with a full neurological examination and demonstrate the neuropathy elsewhere. Remember to state that you would like to perform fundoscopy, examine the abdomen and the rest of the peripheral vascular system, and test the urine for microalbuminuria and proteinuria.

Vascular disorders

CASE 65

🎓 Advanced knowledge

Diabetic feet are caused by neuropathic (microvascular) disease, peripheral (large) vessel disease or superimposed infection.

The aetiology of foot complications in diabetics is varied. They have a poorer lipid profile and a greater prothrombotic tendency than the general population, as well as being more susceptible to infection by *Staphylococcus aureus* and *E. coli*.

Keys to management of the diabetic foot

- Strict foot hygiene
- Meticulous footcare by a chiropodist
- Aggressive treatment of infections, with intravenous antibiotics and debridement where necessary.

CASE 65

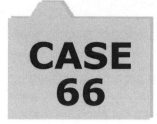

CASE 66

Critical ischaemia

Examine the feet of this patient with rest pain/ulceration.

𝒫 *The examination*

The presence of rest pain/ulceration is indicative of critical ischaemia. Be systematic in your examination, but be aware that the majority of clinical signs occur distally, in the feet and toes. It is crucial that you can take an accurate history of claudication (this may also be examined in an OSCE setting). Look for the following signs:

- Colour

    May be white or dull red
- Trophic changes

    Loss of hair

    Scaly skin

    Gangrenous changes at toes and pressure points
- Ulcers

    As already discussed, arterial ulcers occur in areas that are poorly perfused and at the pressure points. The surrounding skin is cold and the ulcers typically have no granulation tissue. The commonest differential diagnosis is a neuropathic ulcer (the description of ulcers has been dealt with extensively elsewhere)
- Skin temperature

    Compare the two feet
- Capillary refill
- Peripheral pulses

    Radial

    Check the rate and rhythm.

Vascular disorders

CASE 66

Locate the femoral pulses at the mid-inguinal point and compare both sides. Palpate the abdomen for the presence of an aneurysm as you move on to the groin.

Popliteal pulses can be very difficult to feel, and there are a number of acceptable methods. The easiest way is to lie the patient supine, flex the knee slightly and place the thumbs on the tibial tubercle, with the fingers compressing the artery between the two heads of gastrocnemius, against the intercondylar surface of the tibia.

The pedal pulses are very popular with examiners and are best demonstrated bilaterally simultaneously. Stand at the end of the bed, and ask the patient to bring their big toes toward the head. This manoeuvre will make the extensor hallucis longus tendon stand out – the dorsalis pedis pulses are one-third of the way down the foot toward the inter-malleolar line. Without removing your hands, sweep your fingers down to the medial malleolus. Halfway between that point and the calcaneus lies the posterior tibial pulse.

It is wise to auscultate the femoral vessels for bruits.

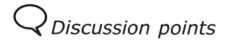 *Discussion points*

These patients are arteriopathic, so remember to examine the rest of the peripheral vascular system and to exclude an abdominal aneurysm.

Be prepared to discuss the manner in which non-invasive and invasive assessment of the vascular system is carried out:

- ankle brachial indices
- duplex ultrasound examination
- angiography.

Vascular disorders

CASE
66

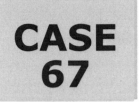

CASE 67

Varicose veins

Examine this man's legs for the presence of varicose veins.

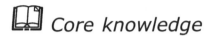 *Core knowledge*

Obtain adequate exposure, but preserve the dignity of the patient. The varicosities may not be the only sign of venous disease. There may also be evidence of venous insufficiency and ulceration.

Lie the patient down and empty the superficial veins. Examine around the ankle, especially the medial side or gaiter area, for the presence of ulcers, venous eczema, lipodermatosclerosis, oedema and atrophie blanche.

Stand the patient up, allowing the veins to fill. Look along the distribution of the long saphenous vein and the short saphenous vein for the presence of varicosities. At the groin, exclude the presence of a saphena varix, which may also have a cough impulse if present.

If varicose veins are confirmed, then you must perform the Trendelenburg test or the tourniquet test. For the former, lie the patient down, elevate the leg to drain the veins and place digital pressure on the sapheno-femoral junction. Then stand the patient up. If the veins do not refill, the sapheno-femoral junction is incompetent. Release the pressure and the veins will fill. If the veins do fill there are distal incompetent perforators, but no information is obtained about the sapheno-femoral junction.

The tourniquet test is similar, but is easier to perform and has the advantage that it can be moved down the leg sequentially to search for the site of the incompetent perforator. The tourniquet test involves applying a tourniquet around the leg at the suspected perforator sites in the leg.

Perthe's test is used to assess the efficacy of the soleal pump. As described previously, empty the veins, applying digital pressure to occlude the sapheno-femoral junction. Then stand the patient up and allow a small amount of blood to fill the distal varicosities. Walk the patient on their toes for a minute, and see whether the veins empty.

Always state that you would examine the abdomen for abdominal or pelvic masses that might be a cause of secondary varicose veins.

Vascular disorders

CASE 67

Q *Discussion points*

Treatment can be non-surgical, involving either the use of graduated compression stockings, or weight loss and exercise.

Surgical treatment includes ligation of the sapheno-femoral junction with stripping and avulsion or avulsion alone. New treatments include subcutaneous endoscopic perforator surgery (SEPS), but no long-term results are available yet.

Vascular disorders

CASE
67

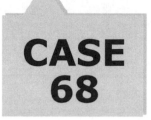

CASE 68

Aortic aneurysms

Examine this man's abdomen for an aneurysm.

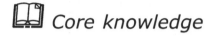 *Core knowledge*

Abdominal aortic aneurysms (AAAs) are the commonest type, occurring in 5% of individuals over 60 years of age according to data from the USA. An aneurysm is defined as a weakness in the arterial wall that results in a dilatation of more than 50% of the normal vessel diameter. The mortality for elective AAA repair is less than 3% in good centres. For those who rupture outside hospital, the mortality rate is 50% if they reach the operating theatre. Mortality is mainly due to blood loss, cardiac arrest, or renal failure and multiple organ dysfunction syndrome (MODS).

The pathophysiology of AAA is that most cases are atherosclerotic, while the rest are inflammatory, mechanical or congenital. The majority (80%) of AAAs are infrarenal, 70% involve the iliac vessels and 20% are associated with other peripheral (eg popliteal) aneurysms. Surgical repair has been shown to be beneficial in patients with aneurysms over 5.5 cm in diameter.

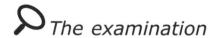 *The examination*

Expose the patient for an abdominal examination, but remember to preserve their dignity.

Inspect

Inspect the abdomen for a mid-line pulsating mass in the epigastrium (remember that the aorta bifurcates at L4 below the umbilicus – do not start too low!), especially in deep inspiration, when it may be easier to see. Are there any previous scars?

Palpate

Begin as you normally would, with superficial and deep palpation. Deep palpation may reveal a mass in the epigastric region. Use your lateral index fingers to estimate the borders of the aneurysm and to demonstrate whether the pulsation is expansile. Expansile masses push the fingers apart, not just up and down. Look for other aneurysms in the femorals and popliteals.

Vascular disorders

CASE 68

Auscultate

Listen over the aorta and the iliac arteries for bruits.

Conclude your examination by stating that you would like to search for concurrent cardiac, carotid and peripheral vascular disease.

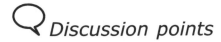

Discussion points

Individuals at risk of AAA development include the following:

- men
- those over 60 years
- smokers
- hypertensive patients
- patients with a strong family history.

Those who should have elective repair include the following:

- symptomatic patients – those with back pain, tender aneurysms or distal embolic events
- patients with aneurysms over 5.5 cm in diameter
- those with aneurysms under 5.5 cm in diameter if they are expanding rapidly (> 1 cm/year).

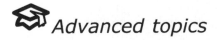

Advanced topics

Endovascular AAA repair is performed with grafts deployed into the aneurysm cavity via a femoral approach by a radiologist and a vascular surgeon. To date, there are no long-term data available on this technique, although papers have been published which suggest that it is associated with better outcomes.

Vascular disorders

CASE 68

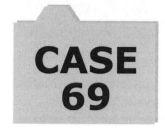

CASE 69

Popliteal aneurysms

Examine this man's legs for aneurysms.

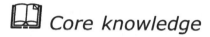 *Core knowledge*

Popliteal and femoral artery aneurysms account for 90% of all peripheral aneurysms, and are almost all degenerative and associated with atherosclerosis. Most are found in association with other aneurysms, and popliteal aneurysms are frequently bilateral. These aneurysms most commonly have a propensity to thrombose, but may also rupture, embolise distally or compress nearby structures.

The examination

Follow the examiner's directions. If you are directed to examine for aneurysms, begin with the femoral pulse, comparing each side. Comment on their presence or absence, their character and whether or not they are normal. Note whether the pulsation is expansile. If it is a popliteal aneurysm, the pulsation is easy to feel and will not need to be compressed against the intercondylar surface of the tibia. You should attempt to gauge the size of the aneurysm. As 50% of popliteal aneurysms are bilateral, examine the other side. If thrombosis has occurred, then the distal pulses may not be palpable.

Remember to tell the examiners that you would like to examine the abdomen for an abdominal aortic aneurysm, and to examine the rest of the limbs for evidence of peripheral vascular disease.

Vascular disorders

CASE 69

Q Discussion points

- About 40% of popliteal aneurysms are asymptomatic.

- Patients with popliteal aneurysms can present with a painful lump behind the knee, or acute or chronic distal limb ischaemia due to embolisation or thrombosis. Only about 10% rupture. Surgical repair may be achieved by simple excision and repair or by venous interposition grafting. For thrombosed aneurysms, pre-operative thrombolysis will lyse thrombosed run-off vessels for potential bypass outflow and improve limb salvage.

- Surgery is indicated for patients with symptomatic aneurysms, aneurysms over 1.8 cm in diameter, and those containing thrombus. Amputation is required in 10–20% of patients who present with acute thrombosis and limb-threatening ischaemia.

Vascular disorders

CASE
69

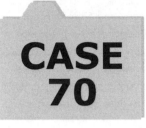

CASE 70

Carotid disease

Examine this man's carotid vessels.

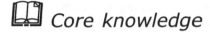 Core knowledge

Carotid bruits occur in 3–4% of the population over 45 years of age, and are found by applying the bell of the stethoscope beneath the angle of the jaw. Aortic valve murmurs radiate into the neck via the carotid arteries and can be mistaken for carotid bruits. Bruits that persist into diastole most probably represent severe carotid disease. A pulsatile mass in the neck that is associated with atherosclerosis, trauma or previous endarterectomy may represent a carotid artery aneurysm.

The examination

Expose the neck as described previously. Proceed directly to auscultation as instructed.

Listen over the course of the common carotid artery, which runs in the anterior triangle of the neck, behind and medial to the sternocleidomastoid muscle (SCM). (Remember to slip the bell of the stethoscope inside the medial border of the SCM while auscultating). The bruit is best heard at end inspiration (hold breath) or during quiet expiration.

Auscultate the praecordium (at the right sternal border, in the second intercostal space) to exclude a transmitted aortic stenosis murmur.

State that you would like to perform a neurological examination looking for residual evidence of a previous cerebrovascular accident (CVA). No long-term clinical signs are seen following a transient ischaemic attack (TIA) or a reversible ischaemic neurological deficit (RIND). You would also need to seek evidence of atherosclerotic disease in the cardiac system, aorta and peripheral vascular system.

Discussion points

Most of the symptoms associated with carotid stenosis or plaques are neurological. As the mortality and morbidity from stroke-related illness are so high, carotid disease is

Vascular disorders

CASE
70

a serious finding. The commonest cause of cerebral events resulting from carotid lesions is cerebral embolisation of either small fragments of degenerated plaque or platelet aggregrates on the plaque surface. An ulcerated lesion is at particular risk for embolisation. The plaque may also cause internal carotid thrombosis, which can be asymptomatic if distal flow is reconstituted via internal ophthalmic collaterals, or it may be devastating if clot propagates or embolises into the middle cerebral artery.

You should be aware by now that the neurological symptoms associated with carotid stenosis are on the contralateral side, and that the amaurosis fugax is on the ipsilateral side. Some of the terms are listed below.

- Transient ischaemic attack (TIA) – a transient hemispheric neurological deficit that may last from several seconds to hours, but not longer than 24 hours. It is characterised by speech, motor and visual disturbances, but there is no lasting deficit. Crescendo TIAs are those that occur in rapid succession with progressively smaller intervals between attacks. They carry a high risk of progression to a permanent neurological deficit.

- Amaurosis fugax – temporary monocular blindness, described as a shade coming down over the eye. It is caused by emboli lodging in the ophthalmic artery. Fundoscopy can demonstrate these cholesterol plaques (known as Hollenhorst plaques) as they traverse the retina.

- Reversible ischaemic neurological deficit (RIND) – a longer-lasting neurological deficit, which can also persist for up to 7 days, but will resolve completely.

- Stroke (cerebrovascular accident) – a permanent neurological deficit that persists for more than 7 days.

Investigation of carotid disease

- Carotid duplex (plaque location, size, ulceration, and the remaining lumen of the internal carotid artery [ICA] / common carotid artery [CCA])
- Carotid angiography (significant stroke risk of around 2%)
- CT/MRI scan of the brain (looking for lacunar-type infarcts).

Surgery for carotid disease

This is indicated in symptomatic patients who have more than 70% stenosis (good evidence from NASCET and ECST trials). Carotid endarterectomy has been demonstrated to produce a sixfold reduction in the rate of stroke at 3 years, with an operative stroke risk of around 2% and an operative mortality rate of 1%. The next commonest complications are haematoma, hypoglossal nerve injury and ipsilateral earlobe numbness.

CASE
70

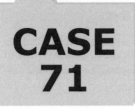

Raynaud's phenomenon

Ask this woman about the colour changes in her hands, and examine them.

The examiner may use a leading question to prompt a spot diagnosis, in this case of Raynaud's phenomenon (RP), and a discussion will then ensue. The original description of RP was of episodic digital ischaemia induced by low temperature or emotion. The classic manifestation of pallor preceding cyanosis and rubor reflects the initial vasospasm, followed by deoxygenation of the static venous blood (cyanosis), and then reactive hyperaemia (rubor) with the return of blood flow. However, the full triphasic colour change is not essential for the diagnosis of RP. (Note the mnemonic: WBC – white, blue, crimson.)

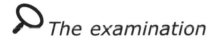 *The examination*

Ask

- What is the main problem with your hands?
- What brings this on?
- Is the weather a factor?
- What are the colour changes?
- Are there any changes with arm or shoulder movements? (To exclude a cervical rib)

Look

- The pathology is usually bilateral.
- There may be ulcers or gangrene on the fingertips.
- In between acute attacks, the skin may be dry and red, and the nails may be brittle.

Vascular disorders

CASE 71

Palpate

- The radial pulse is normal.
- Complete your examination by stating that you would ask about symptoms and look for signs of the secondary causes of Raynaud's phenomenon.

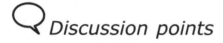 *Discussion points*

The pathophysiology of RP is unknown, but there are several possible causes. They include neurogenic (increased density and sensitivity of α-adrenergic receptors), blood-cell and blood-vessel-wall interactions (activated platelet aggregation, leading to thromboxane A_2 release and increased rigidity of white blood cells and red blood cells causing obstruction of the microcirculation). Alternatively, inflammatory and immunological mechanisms may be responsible, as the most severe cases of RP are seen in association with connective tissue diseases, which are known to have disordered immunological pathways.

The causes of RP may be primary (vasomotor malformation, also known as Raynaud's disease, less severe) or secondary (more severe). There are many secondary causes, including the following:

- blood dyscrasias – polycythaemia
- arterial causes – atherosclerosis, thromboangiitis
- drugs – oral contraceptive pill, α-blockers
- connective tissue disorders
- trauma – vibration (vibration white finger (VWF) disease, or hand arm vibration disorder).

The treatment of RP may be non-surgical (stopping smoking, keeping extremities warm, avoiding predisposing factors), surgical (sympathectomy, amputation if digits are gangrenous) or medical (vasodilators).

Vascular disorders

CASE 71

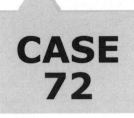

Lymphoedema

Examine this woman's legs.

A diagnosis of lymphoedema is made on the basis of history, physical examination and exclusion of other causes of a swollen limb. It is defined as progressive limb swelling that occurs when the lymphatic system fails to transport fluid via the lymphatics and lymph nodes. Lymphoedema can be classified according to age of onset as follows:

- congenital
- congenital hereditary (Milroy's disease)
- lymphoedema praecox (before the age of 35 years, mostly women affected)
- lymphoedema tarda (after the age of 35 years, no gender difference).

🔍 The examination

Look

- The legs will be grossly swollen, with no particular demarcation.
- It is usually bilateral (unilateral cases are most often due to venous disease).
- Note the loss of contour of the ankle, with a buffalo-hump appearance over the dorsum of the foot.
- There may be lichenified fronds on the toes, and the skin is often thick and indurated (hyperkeratosis, lichenification, peau d'orange).

Palpate

- Is there pitting of the oedema?
- Is there inguinal lymphadenopathy?
- Are there abdominal or pelvic masses?

Vascular disorders

CASE 72

Think

- Is there evidence of congestive cardiac failure?

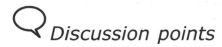

Discussion points

- The other differential diagnoses of lymphoedema are right heart failure, nephrotic syndrome, hypothyroidism and hypoalbuminaemia.

- Secondary (acquired) lymphoedema can be due to neoplastic infiltration of lymph nodes, infections such as *Filaria wucheria bancroftii*, or surgery or radiotherapy.

- Treatment primarily focuses on meticulous foot care, the eradication of infection and elevation. The surgical options include Homans' procedure to debulk the leg, as well as direct lymphovenous anastomosis. These have mixed results and are rarely used.

Vascular disorders

CASE
72

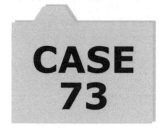

CASE 73

Amputations

Examine this woman's amputation stump.

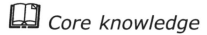

Core knowledge

Amputations may be performed for a variety of reasons, including trauma, resection of malignancy, and peripheral arterial occlusive disease. In most cases, patients who are brought as exam cases are those with amputations due to vascular disease.

Indications for amputation

- Vascular

    Peripheral vascular disease (80–90%)

    Arteriovenous fistulae

    Thromboangiitis obliterans

- Infection

    Osteomyelitis

    Necrotising fasciitis

    Gas gangrene

- Trauma

    Injury

    Burns

    Frostbite

- Malignancy

    Melanoma

    Sarcoma.

For patients with peripheral arterial occlusive disease, the indications are gangrene or persistent painful ischaemia that is not amenable to vascular reconstruction. You should be aware that the survival rate of patients who undergo major amputations is only 50% at 3 years and 30% at 5 years, due to the severe coexistent vascular disease.

Vascular disorders

CASE 73

For exam purposes, the discussion usually focuses on the different types and levels of amputation. The general principles are as follows.

- The level of amputation is determined clinically.
- Reserve as much limb length as possible to aid rehabilitation.
- Remove all of the infected tissue.
- Ensure that there is an adequate blood supply for the stump to heal.

Different types of amputation

- Digital amputations are commonly performed in diabetic patients who are prone to developing osteomyelitis or foot infections.
- Transmetatarsal amputations are performed if several toes are involved in the ischaemic process, or after several digital amputations.
- Below-knee amputations are the most commonly performed type of amputation for patients with severe occlusive arterial disease.
- Above-knee amputations are more difficult to mobilise after surgery, but they heal well.
- Hip disarticulation or hindquarter amputations are rarely performed for peripheral vascular disease.

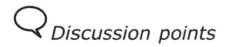 *Discussion points*

Post-operative care

In general, weight bearing is delayed for 4–6 weeks, to allow the stump to mature. Physiotherapy is essential for maintaining limb strength, preventing contracture, and rehabilitating the patient once a prosthesis has been fitted. Some authors advocate the use of stump shrinkers to accelerate the maturation of the stump. As soon as the patient is ready, they should be fitted with a prosthesis and mobilised.

Rehabilitation rates vary widely, but are around 60% and 30% for below-knee and above-knee amputations, respectively. For those with bilateral amputations, the rates drop to around 40% for bilateral below-knee amputation, and 10% for bilateral above-knee amputation. These rates are for patients who can walk without assistance.

Vascular disorders

CASE 73

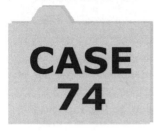

Post-phlebitic limb

Examine this man's legs.

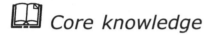 Core knowledge

The post-phlebitic limb is a late consequence of deep vein thrombosis (DVT), and differs from superficial venous insufficiency. It has the appearance of severe skin changes, including lipodermatosclerosis, oedema and varicosities. Although primary varicose veins are due to incompetence of the perforators, it is incompetence of the deep veins from previous DVT which leads to blood flow from deep to superficial veins, causing secondary varicose veins. The results of surgery performed for secondary varicose veins tend to be worse than those of surgery performed for primary varicose veins.

Many DVTs go unnoticed, and consequently the incidence of post-phlebitic limb is high among patients attending for varicose-vein surgery.

The examination

These patients will have the features of chronic venous insufficiency, which are as follows:

- current or healed venous ulcers
- oedema
- lipodermatosclerosis
- haemosiderin deposition
- dilated superficial veins (to return lower limb blood to the inferior vena cava [IVC]).

Vascular disorders

CASE
74

Exclude any arterial disease and confirm that peripheral pulses are present. Then perform Perthe's test, which is used to establish whether the soleal pump is pumping blood effectively out of the veins towards the heart. Place a tourniquet around the thigh, and walk the patient round the examination couch or stationary on the tips of their toes. In normal individuals the deep veins will be patent and allow blood to flow. In patients with deep venous occlusion this is not possible, so the superficial veins will become dilated and the leg will swell.

Discussion points

- The investigation of deep venous occlusion focuses on demonstrating filling defects in the deep veins or showing valvular damage with reflux. This can be achieved with duplex, venography or ambulatory venous pressures.
- Surgery to relieve obstruction of the iliofemoral segments is rarely performed.

Vascular disorders

CASE
74

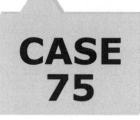

CASE 75

Arteriovenous fistula

Examine this man's right wrist.

The creation of arteriovenous fistulae for the purpose of ensuring intravenous access in patients who require long-term haemodialysis is a common vascular procedure. There may also be patients with congenital or trauma-related arteriovenous malformations, but surgically induced cases are more commonly encountered in short case or OSCE exams.

Expose the patient's arms to the shoulders, as there can also be higher fistulae if there is insufficient systolic pressure at the wrist.

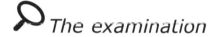 *The examination*

Inspect

- Forearm swelling, usually proximal to the wrist
- Look for previous scars (have other fistulae failed?)
- Describe as for a lump.

Palpate

- The mass is compressible and pulsatile
- There will be a palpable thrill.

Auscultate

- There will be an audible machinery murmur that sounds like a continuous hum.

Most of these patients will have evidence of chronic renal insufficiency, and there may have been previous attempts at fistula formation elsewhere in the arm or in the other wrist. Some of the issues pertaining to this are discussed below.

Vascular disorders

CASE 75

Q Discussion points

The operative technique for the creation of a fistula is via a longitudinal incision at the wrist in the non-dominant forearm, having determined that there is sufficient flow in the radial artery to support the fistula. When the radial artery and cephalic vein have been identified, they are anastomosed via an arteriotomy–venotomy, and the vein is tied off below the fistula. Over the following weeks the high pressure in the arterial system will dilate the cephalic vein, making the fistula suitable for haemodialysis when it is mature. This maturation process can take 5–8 weeks.

The surgeon can also use an ulnar–basilic or brachial–cephalic fistula if necessary. polytetrafluroethylene (PTFE) can also be used if there is distal occlusive arterial disease or if veins are not available.

The advantages of arteriovenous fistulae are as follows:

- high dialyser flow rates
- low infection rates
- long lifespan
- 1-year patency of 90%.

Some of the complications include thrombosis, pseudoaneurysm formation (in the PTFE type), arterial steal syndrome (if there is massive run-off through the fistula, leading to congestive cardiac failure), and sometimes venous hypertension in the hand.

The creation of an arteriovenous fistula generates a hyperdynamic circulation that is manifested as a sinus tachycardia. Cardiac failure occurs if more than 20% of the cardiac output is put through the shunt. When this occurs, the operative treatment is simple – the fistula can be revised or narrowed.

Vascular disorders

**CASE
75**

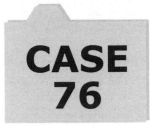

CASE 76

Vascular access devices

Data interpretation.

A variety of vascular access devices are available to OSCE examiners. The placement of these devices is now routine, and they are most commonly used for central access or dialysis access.

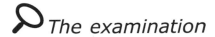

The examination

Central vascular access devices

These are indicated for short- or long-term intravenous infusions.

Short term

- These devices are not tunnelled, and may be in place for days to weeks.
- They are seen in the neck as jugular or subclavian lines, with a double or triple lumen.
- They are inserted using the Seldinger technique, for short-term intravenous infusions or central venous pressure monitoring.
- Subclavian lines are better than jugular lines for comfort and maintenance.

Long term

- These devices are tunnelled, and you will see an exit site and a subcutaneous swelling along the path of the catheter (Hickman/Broviac).
- They can also be left entirely subcutaneously as implanted ports (Portocath).

In addition, there are peripherally inserted central catheters known as PICC lines. These are similar to non-tunnelled lines, and have fewer complications related to insertion.

Vascular disorders

CASE
76

Q Discussion points

Complications of central venous catheters

- Infections
- Thrombosis
- Pneumothorax (50% of cases require a chest drain)
- Haemothorax (guidewire perforates vein, artery or heart)
- Tip migration or malposition (leads to perforation or thrombosis)
- Air embolism
- Catheter compression, fracture or embolisation
- Extravasation of infusate
- Catheter dysfunction.

Vascular access for dialysis has been discussed in the previous case.

Vascular disorders

CASE 76

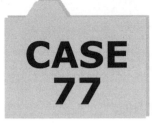

CASE 77

Ulcer – general approach

You are shown a lower limb ulcer.

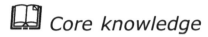

Core knowledge

In many respects the examination is similar to that of a lump, with some additional important points. Decide whether this is a venous, arterial, mixed or neuropathic ulcer on the basis of the clinical findings.

General points

- History – are there symptoms of arterial or venous disease (especially pain or background of diabetes)?
- Inspect the base.

   What colour is it? Is it red or granulating?

   Is there sloughing?

   Is it penetrating into tendon, muscle or bone?

   Is there evidence of malignant change?

   Is there a discharge? If so, is this purulent or bloody?
- Inspect the edge.

   Is it flat or sloping (usually traumatic or a venous ulcer)?

   Is it punched out (usually ischaemic or neuropathic)?

   Is it raised (basal-cell carcinoma)?

   Is it raised and everted (squamous-cell carcinoma)?
- Measure the depth.
- Is there a temperature change?
- Is there any neurovascular deficit in the surrounding area or local muscle groups?

Vascular disorders

CASE 77

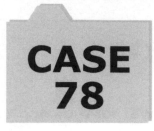

CASE 78

Venous ulcer

Examine this man's leg.

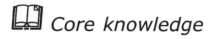

Core knowledge

- Venous ulcers most commonly occur in the gaiter area (the medial aspect of the ankle joint). Ulceration may be precipitated by minor trauma, and is often surrounded by eczema or pigmentation. When accompanied by fibrosis and the brown pigmentation caused by haemosiderin deposition, this is termed lipodermatosclerosis.

- Approximately 80% of patients with lower limb ulceration will have evidence of chronic venous insufficiency, and up to 25% of ulcers will have an arterial cause.

- Venous ulcers are usually shallow with a sloping edge. They vary in size, and there are frequently signs of venous insufficiency. They are often infected and may have a purulent discharge. Varicose veins may also often be found.

- The skin surrounding a venous ulcer is frequently warm, in contrast to the situation in patients with arterial disease, in whom the skin will be cool.

- Peripheral pulses are present in uncomplicated venous disease.

ℚ *Discussion points*

- Venous ulcer usually occurs in conjunction with varicose veins or in the post-phlebitic limb.

- The underlying haemodynamic abnormality in chronic venous insufficiency is venous hypertension.

- Most ulcers heal with conservative treatment. Elevation reduces venous pressure at the ankle to about 15 mmHg, and aids healing. Foot care is also important. Avoid local trauma and be meticulous about hygiene. Four-layer bandages should be considered. These cannot be applied in the presence of arterial disease (an ankle-brachial index (ABI) of > 0.8 is needed). They have a very high success rate, but are not easily tolerated.

- Treatment consists of surgery. If an ulcer does not heal, consider the possibility of malignant change (which can be demonstrated by biopsy). Surgical options include varicose vein surgery and also debridement of the area and split skin grafting.

Vascular disorders

CASE 78

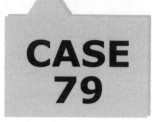

CASE 79

Arterial ulcer

Examine this man's legs.

📖 Core knowledge

- Arterial ulcers are not as common as ulcers secondary to venous disease, and more commonly occur on pressure areas.
- They are usually found on the toes and pressure areas, are usually clean and have a punched-out edge, as there is insufficient blood supply to allow healing to take place. They erode deeply, the base may show exposed tendon or bone, and no granulation tissue will be visible for the reason outlined above. The surrounding skin will be cold, and peripheral pulses will be absent.
- Examine the complete peripheral vascular system.

Discussion points

Causes of arterial ulcers

- Large-vessel disease
    - Atherosclerosis
    - Thromboangiitis obliterans
- Small-vessel disease
    - Diabetes mellitus
    - Polyarteritis nodosa
    - Rheumatoid arthritis.

Vascular disorders

CASE
79

Treatments available

- Offer appropriate analgesia
- Advise the patient on risk factor modification

    Cease smoking

    Obtain good glycaemic control if the patient is diabetic

    Control blood pressure

    Lower lipid levels.

Vascular disorders

CASE 79

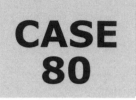

CASE 80

Neuropathic ulcer

Examine this man's leg.

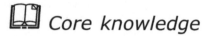 Core knowledge

- The important issue here is to distinguish between arterial and neuropathic ulcers, which can often be difficult.

- Neuropathic ulcers are found on pressure areas, such as the heel, toes and metatarsal heads. They have clean edges, can be very deep, and may often have exposed tendon or bone.

- The key points are that the surrounding skin is of normal colour and temperature, the pulses are all present. but the area may be insensate. These ulcers are painless.

- A history of diabetes in the patient should lead you to suspect a peripheral neuropathy.

- You should finish by performing a complete neurological examination of the cranial and peripheral nerves.

Q Discussion points

Any disease process that can lead to peripheral neuropathy, such as the glove-and-stocking neuropathy that is characteristic of diabetes mellitus, can lead to neuropathic ulcers.

Risk factors for neuropathic ulcers

- Idiopathic causes
- Systemic diseases

  Diabetes mellitus

  Hypothyroidism

  Systemic lupus erythematosus
- Drugs and toxins

  Amiodarone

  Alcohol

  Toxins
- Infections

  Tuberculosis

  HIV

  Leprosy.

Vascular disorders

**CASE
80**

Musculoskeletal disorders

CASE 81

Colles' fracture

This is the X-ray of an elderly woman who has fallen on her outstretched left hand.

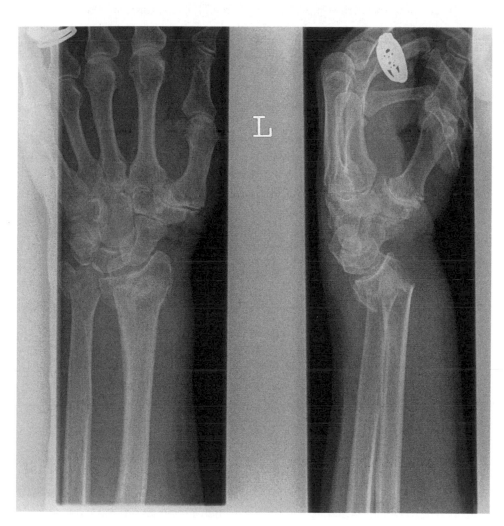

Fig 18

Musculoskeletal disorders

Core knowledge

- This is a Colles' fracture, which is the most common fracture in patients over 40 years of age. Most patients with this fracture are elderly, and they often have osteoporosis.

- This is a distal radius fracture with dorsal angulation and shortening. There is also a radial shift of the fracture fragment.

- Clinically, the patient presents with pain and loss of function. On examination, there may be an obvious dinner-fork deformity with a swollen, tender wrist.

Discussion points

- Treatment usually consists of closed reduction, immobilisation with a plaster cast and rehabilitation. You should have an understanding of the techniques of fracture reduction.

- It is important to be aware of the complications of fractures, such as joint stiffness, non-union and malunion.

Advanced knowledge

- There is a low incidence of carpal tunnel syndrome following Colles' fracture.

- Sudeck's atrophy (a poorly understood condition that is characterised by pain, tingling and weakness in the forearm and hand) may occur after this type of fracture.

CASE 81

CASE 82

Neck of femur fracture

This is the anteroposterior pelvic X-ray of a 70-year-old woman who fell while she was out walking.

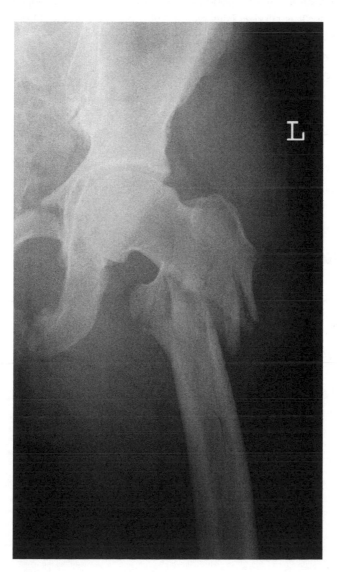

Fig 19

Musculoskeletal disorders

 Core knowledge

- This X-ray shows a fractured neck of femur on the left side. The patient may fall and give a history of feeling the leg give way, or of hearing the fracture. The clinical findings are those of restricted, painful movements, inability to weight bear, and often a shortened, externally rotated leg.

- The X-rays will show a fracture line with the rest of the pelvis and a normal contralateral side. Use Shenton's line to determine the fracture site – that is, whether it is cervical (this can be subcapital, transcervical or basal), intertrochanteric or subtrochanteric.

- The Garden grading system provides information about fracture severity and the degree of displacement between surfaces.

Discussion points

- Medical comorbidity in elderly patients who require surgery.

- Prophylaxis against deep vein thrombosis (DVT) in patients with fractures and immobility.

Advanced knowledge

- The types of fixation include hemiarthroplasty with an uncemented prosthesis such as the Austin–Moore prosthesis or a cemented one such as the Thompson prosthesis.

- A dynamic hip screw may be used to treat basal femoral neck fractures, allowing good functional recovery.

- The hip must be kept in abduction using an abduction pillow for several days to prevent dislocation of the articular surfaces.

CASE 82

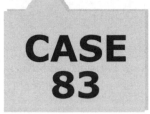

CASE 83

Compartment syndrome

The young man in plaster of Paris underwent intramedullary nailing of a right tibial fracture 24 hours ago. He begins to complain of severe right foot pain. On examination, diminished pedal pulses are found.

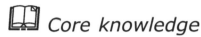

Core knowledge

- This is typical of compartment syndrome. It is an orthopaedic and vascular emergency that is often particularly associated with tibial fractures.

- The clinical findings consist of pain that is out of proportion to what would normally be expected for the injury, and extreme pain on passive stretching. Compartment syndrome is caused by an increase in interstitial fluid pressure within the fascial compartments that is sufficient to compromise the microcirculation and cause myoneural necrosis. The pedal pulses may still be present.

- Tenseness of the compartment on palpation is also a key diagnostic feature, and later on the features of a pulseless limb.

Discussion points

- The diagnosis is confirmed by elevated compartment pressures.

- Treatment consists of fasciotomy of the compartments of the involved muscle group.

Musculoskeletal disorders

🎓 Advanced knowledge

- The common sites for compartment syndrome are the leg following tibial fractures, the forearm following supracondylar humeral fractures, and the foot following calcaneal fractures. The thigh and hand may also be affected after crush injury.

- The compartment pressures in compartment syndrome are of the order of 30 mmHg. This value is distinctly abnormal. As the compartment pressure approaches around 30 mmHg, the microcirculation is compromised.

CASE 83

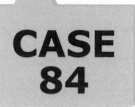

CASE 84

Nerve injuries

You are shown a patient with a nerve injury following a fracture.

Nerve injuries may be introduced by the examiner in a straightforward case of extremity fracture. The common traumatic nerve injuries of the upper limb are listed below. When examining the patient, begin with the hand and work proximally.

 Core knowledge

- Supracondylar humeral fractures, if displaced, and especially in children, can be complicated by entrapment of the radial and median nerves. Compression of the brachial artery may also cause limb ischaemia and compartment syndrome.

- Humeral shaft fractures may have an associated radial nerve (C5–C8) palsy. These generally recover with immobilisation. They are characterised by wrist drop and an insensate area over the anatomical snuffbox, irrespective of the level. There will also be loss of elbow extension as the triceps is affected in high humeral shaft-induced lesions. In addition, they may cause median nerve (C6–T1) palsies, which are manifested by sensory loss in the palmar aspect of the thumb, index, middle and lateral half of the ring fingers.

- An ulnar nerve (C8–T1) palsy is not usually related to trauma of the limbs, but can occur after brachial plexus avulsion. This will give a claw-like appearance to the affected hand, as the ulnar nerve supplies most of the intrinsic hand muscles except for the LOAF muscles (**L**umbricals – lateral two, **O**pponens pollicis, **A**bductor pollicis brevis, **F**lexor Pollicis brevis) innervated by the median nerve.

Musculoskeletal disorders

Discussion points

- These will mainly focus on the clinical demonstrations of each injury.

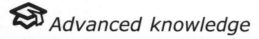

Advanced knowledge

- You may be asked about prevention of joint stiffness and contractures following fracture.
- If a palsy develops after closed reduction, exploration is mandatory as the nerve may be entrapped within the fracture site.

CASE
84

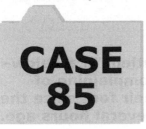

Cervical collar/ advanced trauma life support

You are shown a hard cervical collar.

Musculoskeletal disorders

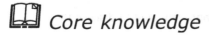 Core knowledge

- These are used to immobilise the cervical spine in patients in whom a neck injury is suspected.
- You should know the ABCDE of the initial primary survey in patients with traumatic injury, namely **A**irway (with cervical spine control), **B**reathing, **C**irculation and control of haemorrhage, **D**isability/neurological deficit, **E**xposure.
- Cervical spine fractures are frequently associated with quadriplegia.

Discussion points

- You should be aware of the importance of the cervical spine X-ray showing all the way to the C7–T1 junction. This is a frequently missed site of injury, as there is a transition from the mobile cervical spine to the immobile thoracic spine.

Advanced knowledge

- The examiner may ask questions about trauma management and the advanced trauma life support (ATLS) protocol.
- The appropriate neurological examination in a patient with suspected spinal injury should include sensory and motor testing of all major muscle groups, with elicitation of the reflexes, as well as a rectal examination and assessment of perirectal sensation.

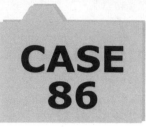

Casts

CASE 86

You are shown a patient in a below-knee cast, who is complaining of excessive pain in their foot since the cast was changed several hours ago.

The issue here is that the cast may be too tight, and you need to discuss the appropriate management of this problem.

 ## Core knowledge

Casts are common, and patients with casts are readily available for examinations.

Describe the cast. What is its anatomical location? Is it complete or is it just a backslab? Remember that the joints on either side of the fracture site should be immobilised to prevent displacement of the fracture.

The complications of casts are listed below.

- The cast may be too tight, due either to poor application or to limb swelling following injury. If there is any evidence of neurovascular compromise remove the cast completely.
- The cast may be too loose, leading to inadequate fixation of the fracture.
- Skin damage may also occur, either on application (due to inadequate padding of pressure points) or on removal (due to damage to the skin caused by instruments).

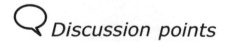 ## Discussion points

Compartment syndrome

This is caused by an increase in the interstitial fluid pressure within the fascial compartments covered by the cast. The clinical findings consist of pain that is out of proportion to what would normally be expected for the injury. Treatment consists of removal of the cast and fasciotomy.

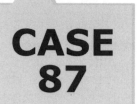

CASE 87

Dupuytren's contracture

Examine the hands of this man who is complaining of loss of function.

This is a palpable and visible contraction of the palmar fascia, most often involving the ring finger. It can be extremely disabling when it is progressive, and is often bilateral. It may also involve the feet. The operative treatment of Dupuytren's contracture is within the domain of orthopaedic or plastic surgeons, although general surgeons sometimes also treat these patients. The condition was first described by Baron Guillaume Dupuytren, a French surgeon.

🔍 The examination

Seat the patient and ask them to place their hands with the palms facing upwards, preferably supported on a pillow.

Inspection of the palmar surface of the affected hand will reveal fixed flexion deformities at both the metacarpophalangeal and proximal interphalangeal joints of the affected fingers. If the condition is severe, the hand may be barely functional and there may be clinical evidence of involvement of the radial side of the hand. There may have been previous hand surgery for this problem, and scars may be visible.

Palpation will reveal a cord-like thickening of the palmar aponeurosis, which is fixed to the skin. Inspect the other hand, and tell the examiner that you would also examine the plantar fascia, as around 5% of patients also have affected feet.

When the condition is incapacitating, the degree of flexion deformity is severe. Ask the patient to move their fingers actively, and then perform passive movement to assess each joint individually.

At the end of the case, you should ask the patient which is their dominant hand and whether they can perform their activities of daily living (ADLs).

Musculoskeletal disorders

Q *Discussion points*

There are many associations with Dupuytren's contracture, including the following:

- idiopathic causes
- alcoholic liver disease
- repetitive trauma associated with manual labour
- familial causes/fibromatoses.

Surgical treatment is reserved for cases with severe functional restriction. This consists of release of the bands via fasciotomy, excision of the palmar fascia with Z-plasty or full-thickness skin grafting, or amputation if the condition is recurrent or unreconstructable. Surgery is usually performed under general anaesthesia with tourniquet control, after exsanguination of the arm. The principal complications are damage to the neurovascular bundle, and recurrence.

The pathogenesis is unclear, but may be related to fibroblast proliferation in response to local tissue ischaemia. This leads to collagen formation with resultant chronic inflammation causing fibrosis.

CASE 87

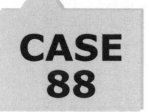

Carpal tunnel syndrome

CASE 88

Examine the hands of this woman who has altered sensation in the thumb and index finger of her left hand.

Carpal tunnel syndrome is caused by compression of the median nerve as it passes through the carpal tunnel. This leads to paraesthesiae in the median nerve distribution, which can be easily reproduced by a number of clinical demonstrations.

The examination

Position the patient as before and expose the arms to the shoulders bilaterally. The clinical signs of carpal tunnel syndrome are predominantly neurological, and it is on this system that you must focus. The problem with demonstrating median nerve signs due to carpal tunnel compression is that more proximal lesions in the route of the nerve can also mimic them.

Inspect for evidence of thenar wasting or previous surgery over the transverse carpal ligament where previous releases may have been performed.

Assess sensory and motor impairment. Compare light touch over the palmar aspects of the thumb and lateral one and half fingers (median nerve) with that of the other fingers. This is a crude method of assessment, but it is aided by the fact that there are certain areas of the digits which are only supplied by one nerve, as listed below:

- median nerve – index and middle fingers, distal phalanges
- ulnar nerve – fifth finger, middle and distal phalanges
- radial nerve – often over the first dorsal interosseus.

Motor assessment involves testing the integrity of the **LOAF** muscles (**L**umbricals – lateral two, **O**pponens pollicis, **A**bductor pollicis brevis, **F**lexor pollicis brevis). Test opposition of the thumb by opposing the thumb and fifth finger and instructing the patient to resist you pulling them apart. The lumbricals are difficult to test reliably. Test abduction of the thumb by placing the dorsum of the patient's hand on a flat surface and instructing her to raise her thumb toward the ceiling against resistance. In the exam, it is probably sufficient to test solely for abduction of the thumb in your motor evaluation.

CASE 88

The small muscles that have a fixed innervation are listed below:

- median nerve – abductor pollicis brevis
- ulnar nerve – palmar interossei (finger adduction)
- radial nerve – metacarpophalangeal extensors (finger extension from the knuckles).

Specific tests

- Tinel's sign is a tingling sensation in the distribution of the median nerve that is induced by tapping over the flexor retinaculum for about 1 minute.
- Phalen's test consists of symptoms induced by manual forced wrist flexion that are relieved by rest.

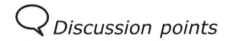

Discussion points

Causes of carpal tunnel syndrome include the following:

- occupational causes (those who work with their wrists flexed)
- rheumatoid arthritis
- idiopathic causes
- diabetes mellitus
- pregnancy
- hypothyroidism
- obesity
- amyloidosis.

The underlying cause of carpal tunnel syndrome is probably nerve ischaemia as increasing pressure occludes the vasa nervorum.

Treatment is either medical or surgical. Medical treatments include local steroid injections to the tunnel, nocturnal splinting of the wrists in a neutral position, and optimisation of any underlying medical cause. Surgical treatment achieves decompression of the carpal tunnel by dividing the flexor retinaculum under tourniquet control. Surgery can be complicated by scar tenderness, failure to relieve symptoms due to inadequate decompression, and nerve injury to the palmar cutaneous nerve or to the motor supply to the small muscles of the thenar eminence.

CASE
88

The use of electromyography (EMG) or nerve conduction studies can differentiate between median nerve lesions higher up and carpal tunnel compression. If the median nerve is disrupted in the arm, the forearm flexors will also be lost, and sensation over the thenar eminence will be affected due to loss of the palmar cutaneous nerve that comes off above the carpal tunnel. EMG will also determine whether this could be due to a brachial plexus or neck lesion. EMG is used to confirm carpal tunnel syndrome prior to surgery.

Musculoskeletal disorders

CASE 88

Hepatobiliary disorders

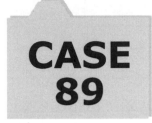

CASE 89

Hepatomegaly

Examine this young man's abdomen.

Obtain adequate exposure and begin to examine the patient's hands, looking for stigmata of chronic liver disease. The examiner may direct you to move straight to the abdominal examination itself.

The common causes of hepatomegaly are listed below:

- Liver metastases
- Alcoholic liver disease
- Myeloproliferative disorders
- Right-sided cardiac failure
- Hepatocellular carcinoma.

The examination

Inspect for stigmata of chronic liver disease.

Hands

- Clubbing (especially with cirrhotic disease)
- Palmar erythema (oestrogen excess)
- Leuconychia (albumin deficiency)
- Dupuytren's contracture
- Liver flap (seen in wrist hyper-extension, advanced liver disease).

Arms and trunk

- Gynaecomastia (subcutaneous enlargement)
- Spider naevi (> 5 is abnormal)
- Scratch marks (pruritus in obstructive jaundice).

CASE
89

Head and neck

- Scleral icterus
- Oral hepatic foetor
- Supraclavicular lymphadenopathy.

Legs

- Pitting oedema.

Inspect the abdomen. There may be generalised abdominal distension secondary to ascites, and in the right upper quadrant there is often the impression of fullness due to hepatomegaly. If there is also portal hypertension, splenomegaly may be present as well as distended abdominal veins, the caput medusae.

Begin palpation in the right iliac fossa, moving your hand proximally during expiration to detect the liver edge, which moves down with inspiration. In your examination, emphasise the fact that you keep your hand static during inspiration and in contact with the skin. Define the hepar in finger breadths from the costal margin, and then palpate it again, noting the consistency and the nature of the edge.

Next percuss upward from below, and then from above downward, to confirm the span. You should be seen to locate the angle of Louis before beginning percussion of the upper border.

After this, auscultate the liver for a bruit, which may sometimes be heard in alcoholic hepatitis and hepatocellular carcinoma, as well as some vascular malformations. Check for splenomegaly (see Case 32) if you suspect portal hypertension (see below), and also check for ascites if there is visible distension (see Case 90). You will not have time to complete a full abdominal examination in an OSCE, but offer this to the examiner.

Portal hypertension

- A portal vein pressure of > 10 mmHg reduces portal blood flow.
- Portal hypertension is usually caused by cirrhosis.
- Intrahepatic causes include schistosomiasis (the primary cause worldwide), right heart failure and infiltration by sarcoid, leukaemia or lymphoma.
- Extrahepatic causes include portal or splenic vein thrombosis.
- The signs are splenomegaly, ascites, venous hum, collateral veins, and caput medusae.

CASE 89

Hepatobiliary disorders

ℚ *Discussion points*

Investigation of the patient with hepatomegaly will consist of liver function tests and coagulation screening (see Cases 98 and 99). Ultrasound examination and CT are the most useful imaging modalities.

It should be noted that in the advanced stages of liver cirrhosis the liver becomes atrophied rather than cirrhotic. Hepatomegaly can also be physiological if it is due to a Riedel's lobe or a hyper-expanded chest (as seen in emphysematous disease).

Hepatobiliary disorders

**CASE
89**

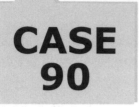

CASE 90

Ascites

Examine the abdomen of this woman who has a previous history of ovarian carcinoma.

The percussion note over the abdomen should be resonant except over the colon, due to bowel gas. Ascites is the accumulation of peritoneal fluid in the abdominal cavity. In early ascites this fluid accumulates in the flanks due to the force of gravity, and a dull percussion note may be detected, known as **shifting dullness**. This requires approximately 2 litres of fluid to be present.

As the amount of fluid increases, a **fluid thrill** may be felt.

☌ The examination

Expose the patient as described previously for an abdominal examination, and conduct a survey for signs of chronic liver disease (see Case 89). Note the distension, which begins at the flanks, leaving the centre flat.

Shifting dullness

Standing on the patient's right side, percuss away from you with your finger in the sagittal plane, moving from the centre to the left flank. Note the point where the note becomes dull. Then roll the patient towards you and percuss again in the same spot. If there is ascites, the note will now be resonant.

Fluid thrill

In more advanced ascites, it will be possible to feel a transmitted thrill. In the exam, use the examiner's hand to prevent transmission through the subcutaneous fat, and flick on the patient's flank with your left hand. Use your right hand on the opposite flank to detect the pulsation.

Finish by performing a full abdominal examination, and tell the examiner that you would look for evidence of congestive cardiac failure and pitting leg or sacral oedema.

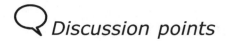 Discussion points

The causes of ascites are defined according to the protein content of the ascitic fluid. If it contains more than 30 grams of protein per litre, it is an exudate. If it contains less than 30 grams per litre, it is a transudate.

Common causes of ascites

- Chronic liver disease (transudate)
- Right-sided cardiac failure (transudate)
- Intra-abdominal malignancy (exudate)
- Hypoalbuminaemia (transudate).

Uncommon causes of ascites

- Lymphatic obstruction (chylous ascites) (exudate)
- Nephrotic syndrome (transudate)
- Infection (tuberculosis) (exudate).

Paracentesis is the removal of ascitic fluid for diagnostic or therapeutic purposes. It can be done at the bedside under aseptic conditions with local anaesthetic and a cannula. If the ascites is loculated or present in small quantities, this procedure can be performed under ultrasound guidance. The fluid is then sent for protein estimation, determination of the presence of malignant cells and microbiological analysis.

In abdominal distension due to ascites there will be flank fullness, and the umbilicus will point downward and may also be everted.

Hepatobiliary disorders

CASE
90

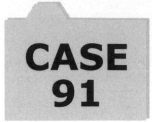

Surgical jaundice

Describe the causes of the condition and appropriate management of this 75-year-old woman who presents with jaundice.

CASE 91

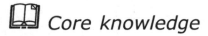

Core knowledge

Pre-hepatic

This is often due to haemolysis (think of patients with severe sepsis, and also following blood transfusions).

Hepatic causes

Think of diseases that affect the parenchyma, such as hepatitis and cirrhosis. Also consider hepatocellular carcinoma or metastatic liver disease from another source. Finally, consider drugs that can cause parenchymal liver damage.

Post-hepatic (obstructive)

This is commonly referred to as surgical jaundice. It is most often seen in patients with gallbladder disease where stones block the common bile duct. It is also seen in patients with carcinoma of the pancreas or bile ducts, or where there are involved lymph nodes compressing the bile ducts.

Questions to ask

- Do you have dark urine/pale stools?
- Does your skin itch?
- Have you had a blood transfusion in the past?
- Are you taking any new medications?
- What is your alcohol intake?
- Have you been abroad recently?

Possible benign cause

- Have you ever had gallstones?
- Do you suffer from colicky abdominal pain after meals?

Possible malignant cause

- Have you been unwell for a long time?
- Have you had any weight loss or decrease in appetite?
- Has there been a change in your bowel habit?
- Do you suffer from pain in your back or abdomen?

Discussion points

- How to interpret liver function tests showing an obstructive pattern (elevated alkaline phosphatase, total bilirubin), hepatocellular pattern (elevated alanine aminotransferase, aspartate aminotransferase) or mixed pattern.
- The treatment of common complications of gallstone disease, and the operative and palliative treatment of pancreatic malignancy.
- The use of common investigations such as liver ultrasound, liver biopsy and endoscopic retrograde cholangio-pancreatography (ERCP).

Advanced knowledge

- Advances in treatment, such as biliary stenting of malignant strictures.
- Advances in diagnosis, such as magnetic resonance cholengio-pancreatography (MRCP) (non-invasive diagnostic imaging of the biliary tree using MRI without contrast).

Hepatobiliary disorders

CASE
91

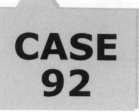

Biliary colic

CASE 92

Describe the appropriate management of a 48-year-old woman who presents with severe right upper quadrant pain and vomiting.

This sounds like gallbladder pathology.

Core knowledge

Differential diagnosis

- Biliary colic
- Acute cholecystitis
- Peptic ulcer disease
- Pancreatitis.

Essential investigations

- Ultrasound abdomen
- Gastroscopy
- Liver function tests
- Amylase.

Important clinical signs

- Murphy's sign (in cholecystitis, cessation of inspiration with pressure on the tip of the right ninth costal cartilage, that is not present on the left)
- Boa's sign (in biliary colic, the patient may complain of right scapular tip paraesthesia)
- Cullen's sign and Gray–Turner's sign (both in acute haemorrhagic pancreatitis, periumbilical or flank discoloration due to tracking of retroperitoneal blood).

CASE
92

ℚ *Discussion points*

Ultrasound examination is useful for detecting calculi, gallbladder wall oedema and fluid around the gallbladder. Compare it with CT, which is useful for demonstrating dilated bile ducts as well as lesions of the liver and pancreas. It is also helpful for evaluating the bowel and retroperitoneum in the diagnosis of abdominal pain.

The aetiology of gallstones, which are due to precipitation of cholesterol in supersaturated bile. Most (around 70%) are mixed cholesterol stones, the remainder consisting of pure pigment or calcium bilirubinate.

Complications of stone disease include the following:

- jaundice
- pancreatitis
- cholecystoduodenal fistulae
- gallstone ileus.

🎓 *Advanced knowledge*

- Gallbladder carcinoma – rare (found in 0.25% of cholecystectomies)
- Delayed vs immediate cholecystectomy – surgery can be undertaken during the same admission or 6 weeks later
- Conversion criteria from laparoscopic to open cholecystectomy (where anatomy is unclear; dissection is unsafe, usually secondary to adhesion).

Hepatobiliary disorders

**CASE
92**

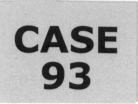

Ascending cholangitis

CASE 93

Describe the differential diagnosis of an 80-year-old man who has a 4-day history of severe right upper quadrant pain, with jaundice, rigors and dehydration.

📖 Core knowledge

- It is important to recognise this as ascending cholangitis, which is a medical emergency. This topic may be introduced by the examiner in relation to a case of acute cholecystitis or some other straightforward biliary case.

- Charcot's triad consists of jaundice, rigors and right upper quadrant pain.

- Associated clinical signs include intermittent pyrexia and tender hepatomegaly.

- This is an ascending infection of the biliary tract, and is commonly associated with bile duct obstruction due to stones. You may also be asked about the management of retained common bile duct stones. These may be identified on ultrasound or MRI, and can be extracted either at endoscopic retrograde cholangio-pancreatography (ERCP) or during open surgery.

❓ Discussion points

- Interpretation of the clinical and investigative findings (positive blood cultures, obstructive liver function tests, dilated intrahepatic bile ducts on ultrasound examination).

- What is the best antibiotic therapy for this disorder and why? (It is usually caused by *E. coli*.)

🎓 Advanced knowledge

- Methods of endoscopic or percutaneous bile drainage.

CASE 94

Data – Endoscopic retrograde cholangio-pancreatography (ERCP)

This is an ERCP picture showing a stricture of the lower end of the common bile duct. What are the possible causes of this stricture? Are there any other means of imaging it which could be employed here?

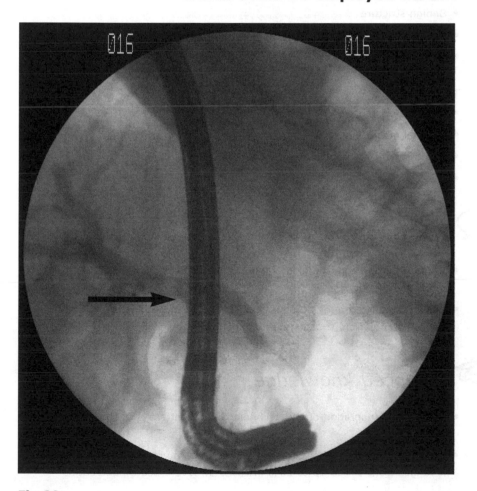

Fig 20

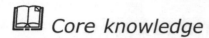 *Core knowledge*

ERCP

- How is it done? By using endoscopy and radiological imaging
- What is the pre-operative work-up? Consent, coagulation screen and platelet count
- What are the complications? Pancreatis and bleeding

Biliary strictures

Causes
- Benign stricture
- Primary sclerosing cholangitis
- Malignant stricture.

Treatment
- Depends on cause
- Internal biliary bypass
- Stenting for external biliary drainage.
- Resection

Discussion points

- Is ERCP more diagnostic or therapeutic? (With the advent of MRCP, it is now more therapeutic.)
- What is sphincterotomy? (Endoscopic cutting of the sphincter of Oddi to release stones from the common bile duct.)

Advanced knowledge

- MRCP is an adaptation of MRI technology. No contrast is used, and it is non-invasive.
- The main complication of ERCP is pancreatitis. The mortality associated with it ranges from 1% to up to 20% in cases of severe acute pancreatitis.

CASE 94

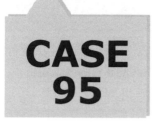

Data – biliary stents and drains

Describe these devices (external biliary stent/T-tube) and what they are used for.

📖 Core knowledge

- These devices are used to treat bile duct obstruction. External biliary drains may be used to drain bile in the presence of strictures (secondary to either inflammation or malignancy), prior to definitive treatment.

- T-tubes are latex tubes that are often placed in the common bile duct after common bile duct exploration. The tube is brought out through the skin, and bile drains into a bag at the bedside. You will be asked to comment on the quantity and nature of the bile.

- Make sure that you know about the management of T-tubes, when they should be clamped, and what it means if the patient develops pain or jaundice. T-tubes are inserted following bile duct exploration, and the duct is then closed over them. They are less commonly seen now in surgical wards. At 10 days after surgery, a T-tube cholangiogram is performed to confirm that there is free flow of bile to the duodenum. The tube is then withdrawn.

Discussion points

- Which patients require common bile duct exploration at cholecystectomy? Most patients can have common bile duct stones removed at endoscopic retrograde cholangio-pancreatography (ERCP). Those in whom this is impossible may require open exploration.

- What is cholangiography and how is it performed? Cholangiography was commonly used during cholecystectomy prior to the development of ERCP to outline the anatomy of the extrahepatic biliary tree. Radio-opaque contrast was injected into the cystic duct prior to removal of the gallbladder. Cholangiography confirms normal anatomy and demonstrates stones in the ducts, which can then be removed.

- What neoplasms commonly cause extrahepatic bile duct obstruction? Commonly, these neoplasms are pancreatic carcinoma and cholangiocarcinoma. In rare cases, lymphoma may cause extrinsic compression of bile ducts from enlarged nodes.

Advanced knowledge

- What are the uses and complications of bile duct stenting?

CASE
95

CASE 96

Data – liver metastases

A CT scan of the abdomen of a woman who is complaining of mild upper abdominal pain demonstrates multiple hepatic deposits. She has a background of node-positive breast cancer, which was treated by left wide local excision and axillary clearance followed by adjuvant chemotherapy and radiotherapy 5 years previously. How would you manage this woman's clinical situation?

Hepatobiliary disorders

 Core knowledge

- This patient has metastatic liver disease. You should be able to recognise obvious disease on a CT scan and correlate this with liver function tests.

- Make sure that you know the difference between curative and palliative surgery (palliative surgery is for the relief of symptoms).

- Broadly describe the adjuvant treatments that are available for this patient.

Discussion points

- Ultrasound and guided liver biopsy

- The concept of staging patients with cancer.

- The liver as a site of tumour deposition. Why do certain malignancies not spread to that site?

Advanced knowledge

- What are the treatment options for patients with liver metastases confined to one lobe of the liver?

- Discuss the optimum investigations for re-staging patients with solid tumours who present with distant metastases (CT/PET scanning/isotope bone scan).

CASE 96

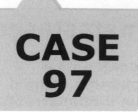

CASE 97

Data – pancreatic carcinoma

A CT scan of a 44-year-old man who presented with painless jaundice which is rapidly progressing in intensity demonstrates a mass in the head of the pancreas. He also had a palpable gallbladder on examination.

 Core knowledge

- Aetiology of pancreatic carcinoma – it is associated with smoking, caffeine, diabetes and asbestos exposure. The disease is more common in patients with chronic pancreatitis.
- General knowledge of the operative treatment – palliative procedures (to drain bile, relieve gastric outlet obstruction or relieve jaundice) are more commonly performed than curative pancreaticoduodenectomy (Whipple's operation).
- Significance of a palpable gallbladder – Courvoisier's law (a palpable gallbladder in the presence of jaundice is rarely due to stones).

Discussion points

- Prognosis of pancreatic cancer
- Courvoisier's law and its importance

Advanced knowledge

- Whipple's operation
- Palliative procedures for biliary bypass

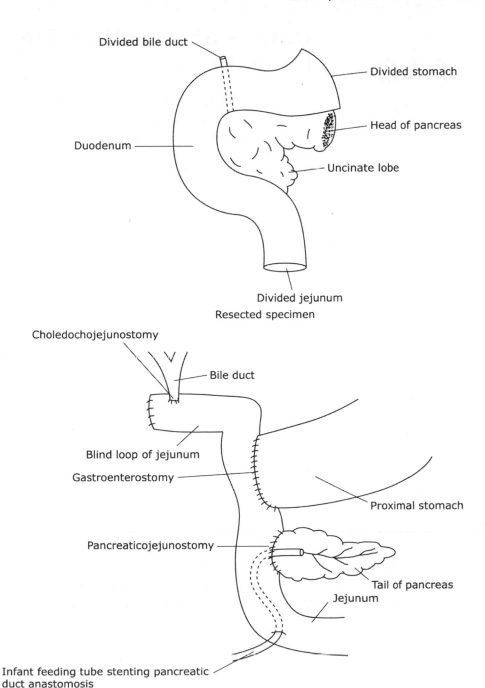

Fig 21 Whipple's procedure

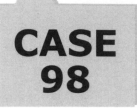

CASE 98

Data – obstructive liver function tests

These are the liver function test results for a 66-year-old heavy smoker who has presented with jaundice and weight loss. Comment on their significance and possible causes.

Hepatobiliary disorders

		Normal values
Aspartate aminotransferase (AST)	43 iu/l	1–50
Alanine aminotransferase (ALT)	54 iu/l	1–50
Total bilirubin	413 μmol/l	1–21
Alkaline phosphatase	380 iu/l	30–110
γ-Glutamyl transferase	76 iu/l	1–35
Amylase	227 iu/l	25–125

 ## Core knowledge

- This is an obstructive pattern of liver function derangement.
- Other tests that you could perform to determine hepatic function include coagulation profile, albumin levels and liver biopsy.

Discussion points

- The hyperamylasaemia in this patient is non specific.
- The best places to demonstrate clinical jaundice are the eyes and skin, because bilrubin is deposited in the elastin fibres. Scleral jaundice is more obvious than skin jaundice.

🎓 Advanced knowledge

AST and ALT sometimes become elevated in mainly obstructive jaundice, due to hepatocyte damage following prolonged periods of bile duct obstruction.

The relative advantages of each imaging modality in the jaundiced patient are as follows.

- Ultrasound – non-invasive, more useful for biliary abnormalities and stones than for the pancreas
- CT scan – excellent for liver, pancreas and nodal enlargement
- ERCP – therapeutic, but associated with complications
- MRCP – non-invasive, but diagnostic only.

Hepatobiliary disorders

CASE
98

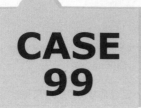

Data – hepatocellular liver function tests

CASE 99

These are the liver function test results for a 35-year-old man who has presented with jaundice, weight loss and gross ascites. Comment on their significance and likely causes.

		Normal values
Aspartate aminotransferase (AST)	4300 iu/l	1–50
Alanine aminotransferase (ALT)	5499 u/l	1–50
Total bilirubin	113 μmol/l	1–21
Alkaline phosphatase	380 iu/l	30–110
γ-Glutamyl transferase	760 iu/l	1–35
Amylase	1278 iu/l	25–125

 ## Core knowledge

This patient has hepatic failure.

The common causes include the following:

- cirrhosis
- drugs (halothane)
- viral hepatitis
- paracetomol overdose
- non-steroidal anti-inflammatory drugs
- poisoning.

It is important to be aware of the functions of the normal liver, which include the following:

- synthesis of clotting factors
- pH balance and urea metabolism
- drug and hormone metabolism
- removal of gut endotoxins
- production of bile.

CASE 99

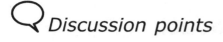Discussion points

- The neurological sequelae of acute and chronic hepatic failure – hepatic encephalopathy, a metabolic neuropathy of uncertain cause, but probably related to failure of the liver to eliminate gut toxins, as well as the accumulation of ammonia, which crosses the blood–brain barrier.

Advanced knowledge

- Make sure that you know the criteria for and role of orthotopic liver transplantation. In children, this procedure is usually undertaken for cirrhosis or metabolic disorders. In adults, it is commonly performed for primary biliary cirrhosis, chronic active hepatitis or metabolic disorders.

Hepatobiliary disorders

CASE 99

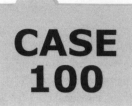

CASE 100

Data – acute pancreatitis

These are the Imrie–Glasgow criteria for a 57-year-old woman who presented with severe abdominal pain associated with a recent alcohol binge. What do these results indicate and how would you grade the severity of her illness?

		Normal values
Age	57 years	
Albumin	29 g/l	35–50 g/l
White blood count	18 x 10^9/l	3.5–11/l
Calcium	1.7 mM/l	2.1–2.6 mM/l
Glucose	16 mM/l	<11.1mM/l
PaO$_2$	9 kPa	10–11.3 kPa

 Core knowledge

- Severe acute pancreatitis is an illness of acute onset characterised by upper abdominal pain and variable clinical findings ranging from mild abdominal tenderness to rebound tenderness. An acute attack may also be associated with vomiting, fever, tachycardia, leukocytosis and an elevated blood or urine amylase.

- Amylase is not a sensitive indicator of organ damage.

- Pancreatitis is classified as either acute or chronic.

✑ *Discussion points*

- Causes of acute pancreatitis (gallstones, alcohol, idiopathic).

- The majority of patients will improve with conservative management and supportive treatment by eliminating oral intake and ensuring adequate hydration and analgesia.

- Surgery may have a role in those patients with pancreatitis who are deteriorating. Removal of necrotic pancreatic tissue by interventional radiology techniques or open surgery is advocated by some authors, but the benefits of this are unclear.

🎓 *Advanced knowledge*

- Complications of pancreatitis can be anticipated if the patient is worsening clinically. Diagnosis is by repeat CT scanning. Patients with severe forms of the disease may develop multi-organ failure.

- With regard to the management of pancreatic pseudocysts, if the patient is asymptomatic, leave them alone. Otherwise, they can be drained percutaneously.

Hepatobiliary disorders

CASE 100

Index